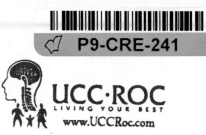

Wake Up, Humans!

The Chiropractic Principle That Restores the Body's Innate Healing Power, Transforms Lives, and Unlocks Human Purpose

Dr. Steve Judson

Editorial project management: Corey McCullough, cbmcediting.com
Printed in the United States of America

FIRST EDITION

ISBN: 978-09966902-6-3 (international trade paper edition)
ISBN: 978-0-9966902-7-0 (e-book edition)

Published by Stephen Judson
10 9 8 7 6 5 4 3 2 1

Dedication

This book is dedicated to my mom and dad. Without you, I wouldn't be here. Thank you for guiding me and showing me the meaning of strength.

To my amazing sister Kristene for always being there and being a rock.

To my brother Ronnie for his sacrifice that he did not choose.

To the Creator for my vision to change millions of lives.

To my college fraternity brothers for showing me a different way of life and how to be a better man—particularly Chris Muldoon and John Seery. Back when I never could afford my rent or my train ticket to get into the city for school, you guys were there. You are a massive part of my success today.

To my staff at Judson Family Chiropractic over the years, including but not limited to Larissa, Elycia, Cindy, Ruthie, Jenn, and Kathy. Without these incredible people, everything would have fallen apart.

To my amazing crew at Dynamic Essentials (there are too many of you to name) and in Chiropractic Bands of Brothers all around the world, especially my Connecticut Band of Brothers. I love and appreciate you.

To Eddie Martinez, Brian Lieberman, Peter Amlinger, Drew Henderson, Lucas Matlock, Anna Hughes, Johnny Balsamo, Jim Sigafoose, and Michael Kale. And to Dr. Sid E. Williams for teaching me the lasting purpose mindset and guiding me on this path.

To all my reviewers, including Rocco Crapis, Megan Afshar, Mike Buonapane, Meghan Dubaldo, and Diane Adams for your help and feedback.

To Corey McCullough for all your hard working managing this project, holding me accountable, and getting shit done.

To my patients, for trusting me through the years.

Most importantly, to my five kids who I adore and who have taught me how to love beyond measure, and to my wife Tammy for being my rock, always standing by my side, and putting up with all my craziness in my mission to make massive change in the world. I love you.

Contents

Preface: A Disclaimer about This Book 6

Prepare to Be Healed 8

My Mission 10

How's Your Atlas? 12

Chapter 1: Judson 101: The Forgotten Truth of Human Healing ... 14

Vertebral Misalignments 16

The Chiropractic Adjustment and Living Clear 17

The Fundamental Truths of Human Health 18

The Chiropractic Chemistry of Life 19

What Do Chiropractors Do? 26

Chapter 2: My Story 32

The Day Ronnie Judson's Life Was Stolen 34

"I Don't Know What's Wrong with Me" 35

What the Heck is a Chiropractor? 38

This Is Life Now 39

Chapter 3: Dynamic Essentials: My Call to Chiropractic 44

The Dynamic Essentials of Health 46

The History of Chiropractic 48

The Vertebral Subluxation: The Root of Human Dis-ease 51

Dr. B.J. Palmer's Law of Life 53

Chapter 4: A Deeper Look at Chiropractic 58

The Nervous System 59

Reduced Nerve Flow Equals Reduced Body Function 63

The Cause of Vertebral Subluxations 65

The Atlas: The Key to Human Health 67

What Does a Chiropractic Adjustment Do? 68

Chapter 5: Innate Power 74

Innate Intelligence: The Process of Life 75

Ease and Dis-ease 77

Paralysis of Action: The Process of Death 78

Chapter 6: Retracing: The Journey Continues 82

Chiropractic Fails Ronnie Judson . . . Again.............................. 83
Momentum and Retracing 86

Chapter 7: The Symptom Mentality and the Folly of Drugs..........90
A World Without Drugs... 92
Health Care vs. Sick-Care 94
Ronnie Judson Today.. 96
Are You Subluxated?... 98

Chapter 8: Uncompromising: The Chiropractic Principle............102
A Failure Story 106
Incongruent: The Rise of Unprincipled Chiropractic................... 108
Avoid the Mixers..110
Look Within: Shed Your Husk 113
Write Your Own Story..116

Chapter 9: Love and "Miracle" Stories 120
Tommy's Story.. 122
A Research Story... 128
Love Your Kids.. 130

Chapter 10: Running from God 140
Iron Men 141
Something's Not Right... 143
That Face Doctors Make... 144
The Flight Is Full.. 148
When We Are at Our Worst... 151

Chapter 11: Living On-Purpose.. 154
Know Your Mission.. 155
Purpose and Peace.. 160
The Shit Is Never Far from the Fan 162

Chapter 12: The Genius of Living Innately 166
Our Far-Reaching Thoughts and Actions................................. 170
"I Can't See a Chiropractor Because. . . .".............................171
How to Find a Principled Chiropractor..................................173
Wake Up!...174

Appendix 178

Preface

A Disclaimer about This Book

There is only one way to start this book, and that is to give credit where credit is due. Without the Lord in my life, I wouldn't be where I am. I never would have achieved any of the things I have today, and I certainly wouldn't have overcome all the challenges that threatened to disrupt my journey. I realize there are other people in this world who are called to overcome many more hardships than I ever had to face, but in my life, my faith in Jesus is what has pulled me through it all. It molded me into the man who shares these words with you today.

The three Bible verses I most treasure are Philippians 4:13: "I can do all things through Christ who strengthens me." That verse is literally tattooed on my arm. My other favorite verse is John 3:16. You've probably heard that one before because it's one of the most quoted verses in the Bible: "For God so loved the world that He gave His only begotten Son, that whoever believes in Him should not perish but have everlasting life."

But another verse that has stuck with me for years and helped me find my voice occurs in Matthew 21:12. This is one you don't hear about so much. . . .

To be clear, you don't have to be a person of faith to receive the message in this book. Some people believe in God. Some have faith in the Universe or the Source. Others are atheists or agnostics. Regardless of what you believe, we can all learn a lesson from Jesus about how to love people. Love was the chief aim of his ministry. He traveled around teaching people and loving people—hugging them, kissing them, serving them, washing their feet, and healing them. But in Matthew 21:12, we see a different side of Jesus; we see the unapologetic wrath of the Lord.

Jesus enters the temple in Jerusalem. This was a place intended as holy ground, but immoral men had turned the temple courts into a marketplace, selling goods for their own profit, deceiving for the sake of financial gain, and disgracing his father's house. Jesus became enraged. He didn't ask them to leave. Instead, he flipped over their tables. The book of John even says he made a whip of cords to drive the men out. He forcibly, violently drove the corruption out of his temple.

If you've never heard that story before, it might be a bit shocking. Flipping tables? Driving people out with whips? The truth is, Jesus was not the meek, mild-mannered lamb he is made out to be. He was pure love. And his love could be as fierce as a lion.

The title of this book, *Wake Up, Humans!* is not a polite request. It is an order. It is an imperative command. It might even sound kind of harsh, and I will warn you now, *a lot* of the content of this book is going to come off as harsh. My words come from a place of love, and at times, you might find them a little abrasive, a little scathing, and sometimes even convicting. That is because we cannot solve a problem with the same mindset that created it, nor can I share the solution in the same voice that created the problem. Be prepared to be challenged and to hear some things you have never heard before.

When the situation called for it, Jesus, the man who taught people to turn the other cheek, became a warrior ready to fight for what he believed in—unwilling to tolerate what he took to be an offense against the sanctity of holy ground. Your body is holy ground. It is a temple. To experience true healing, you must take active steps to keep it clear, and drive out the corruption. You already possess all the tools you need to do that. In this book, I simply teach you how to use them.

This book is pure love, but sometimes love is a left hook. I am not known for being a man who pulls punches, and I don't intend to do it here. This is a real, candid conversation. I speak from the heart, left hooks and all.

Don't say I didn't warn you.

Prepare to Be Healed

Your body can heal itself.

Pause for a second. Reread those words and let the awesome truth of that statement sink in. Think about how amazing that is. *Your body can heal itself.* That is incredible.

It shouldn't really be a shocking concept. We all inherently know the human body heals itself. But for some reason, we like to convince ourselves that medicine does the healing, not the body. The truth is, medicine doesn't heal you. In fact, 100 percent of healing is done within the body using its own power.

Your body knows everything it needs to know the moment you enter this world, and it can do everything it needs to do, all on its own, without anyone's help. There is a blueprint within you that tells your body how to go about its daily processes, including healing. Healing is innate. You currently contain all the mechanisms that will ever be needed to heal yourself of anything. The problem is, certain interferences sometimes disrupt these processes, which leads to reduced health in the body.

Many people would be shocked to learn that the paradigm of human health they have believed all their lives is based on a fallacy. You might also be shocked to learn that the innate nature of healing is the core philosophy of **THE PRINCIPLE OF CHIROPRACTIC.**

When most people hear the word "chiropractor," they think *back pain*. We fix stiff necks, right? We crack backs. Speaking as a chiropractor, I can tell you there is nothing we hate more than being called "back crackers," but I'll admit, I used to be guilty of the same ignorance. When I was growing up, I didn't even know what chiropractic was. That's part of what makes my story so remarkable and, in a way, unlikely.

I wish I could tell you I learned about chiropractic from someone who reached out to my family and cared for us when we needed it most. Instead, my introduction to chiropractic was rooted in tragedy.

My older brother Ronnie Judson was a miraculous kid whose life was changed forever after he sustained a neck injury during a standard college football practice. In the following years, he was diagnosed with multiple mental disorders and soon ended up in a psychiatric hospital—the first of many. Ronnie's life became an endless cycle of pain and suffering, and all I could do was watch and wish something could be done to save him.

Imagine my surprise, years later, to learn there was.

True chiropractic is based on the central nervous system and a little bone called **THE ATLAS.** Most people do not know that chiropractic care has the potential to wake up humans and restore the body's innate healing power. When I learned this for myself, I wondered, "Why didn't anyone tell my family about this sooner? Why have I never heard any of this stuff before?"

To this day, so many people ask me the same question when they come into my chiropractic office and learn for the first time about **LIVING CLEAR** through chiropractic care. "Why have I never heard this before?" It is a tragedy that must stop, and it is the reason this book is in your hands. Too many of us are asleep, unaware of an incredible truth that could literally save our lives if we only understood its power.

My chiropractic practice started as a tiny, one-room office in a run-down, rented old house. Today, I am the owner and operator of Judson Family Chiropractic, a high-volume practice run out of a 10,000-square-foot facility in Newington, Connecticut. I have a beautiful family with an amazing wife and five incredible kids. I am also a regular speaker at chiropractic and health events across the country. Given everything I have learned over the years and have seen with my own eyes, I believe we humans possess everything we need to help us adapt to the environment, heal from anything, and make our lives nearly perfect—to make life abundant, whole, and full. It all comes from within, and as long as nothing interferes with our expression of life, life will be awesome.

My Mission

It's difficult for me to define the book in your hands. As a younger man, I never would have guessed I would become a chiropractor, let alone write a book. Back then, my dream was to be a professional baseball player. In high school, I actually had professional teams looking at me. I was a pitcher. But then I tore my rotator cuff, I couldn't pitch anymore, and all those dreams vanished.

I had job offers on Wall Street, but I didn't want to do that. It was what my father had done, and I hated it. Instead, I went to college and became an English major because it came naturally to me, but I had no idea what I wanted to do with my life. At the end of my junior year, I discovered this thing called chiropractic, and the rest is history.

I'm not just a chiropractor. I'm a **PRINCIPLED** chiropractor. (You'll soon understand what that means and how to tell the difference between principled and unprincipled chiropractors.) My focus is not just on providing care for my patients but educating the masses about the truth of chiropractic.

People sometimes ask me what I talk about when I speak at events, but all I can tell you is that I get up onstage, say a prayer, and let it rip, and things come through. People travel long distances to listen to my talks. Friends, colleagues, and patients call me late at night to discuss their problems when no one else will listen to them. Patients even ask me to officiate their wedding ceremonies. Through it all, I do my best to guide these people through emotional and spiritual pain. It blows me away when people tell me I've transformed their lives, awakened them to their purpose, changed their marriage or their relationship with their kids, made them stop drinking, prevented them from committing suicide. . . . But that's not me. It's **LIFE**. I'm just trying to be a servant of the source. That's what gets results. And that's what I want to share with people.

New patients come into my office all the time, people in their twenties, who have shockingly weak expressions of life. Many humans' nervous systems have been under constant, unseen, devastating pressure since the day they were born (see Chapter Four). When a patient finally understands how the body heals, it wakes up a giant within them. I travel across the country and around the world, speaking at events, all in the hopes of waking up giants wherever I go. Now, it's your turn.

Live free. Have faith. Love life. Kick ass. Be **ABUNDANT**.

My mission is as follows: With reckless abandon, I serve others by helping them through their pain. I do it in a loving, hardcore, in-your-face way. In this book, you'll get the real me. Nothing else. At its core, this book is an educational tool about chiropractic care, but it's also a resource for anyone looking to increase their quality of life physically, emotionally, and spiritually.

I have learned that a lot of difficult times come hand-in-hand with the good times. I've been knocked down and beaten up. There have been moments when I've stared death in the face and yet somehow knew everything would be okay. I've been through a lot of shit, but that shit created my life and made me who I am.

I hope this book will prove to you that if we can tap into the principles of living clear, creating a mindset for success, and cultivating a core group of people who love us, we can rebound from the down times. Every man, woman, and child goes through these things. This book is to help them realize they are not alone and to show them a better way of life—to help them discover their inborn ability to heal.

I want people in all stages of life to realize that all their answers truly can come from within. God gave us all the resources. Whether it means healing physical or emotional wounds, the answers will come from within. Have faith in a few life principles, and you will realize you can get through anything.

How's Your Atlas?

I have often said we could change the entire world if people understood one simple question: "**HOW'S YOUR ATLAS?**"

In this book, you will learn that if your atlas is clear, and if you take certain action steps and believe in yourself and the power that made you, *anything* in life is possible.

I know it sounds cliché to say "anything is possible," but that's only because the awesome truth of that statement has been diluted by halfhearted repetition. If you can learn to live clear and look within, the right answers will come to you. You are equipped for that—we're all equipped for that. It's just a natural law.

My mission is to **WAKE UP HUMANS** to this incredible truth. So right here at the beginning of this book, you will relearn everything you thought you knew about how the body works.

Again, this message might sometimes be difficult to hear. Everyone needs to receive it, but not all are ready for it. If you are not willing to challenge some preexisting notions about human health and reevaluate how you live your life in order to discover the truth—if you aren't willing to *wake up*—then you might as well put this book down right now. Put it aside. Someday, when you are ready, you'll be drawn back to it, and it will be waiting for you.

Every book I read changes me in some way. My goal is for this book to change you by catapulting your life in a new, positive direction. My message will either frustrate you, or it will enlighten you and make you better; there is no in between.

Either way, when you finish reading this book, you will be a different human being.

Chapter 1

Judson 101: The Forgotten Truth of Human Healing

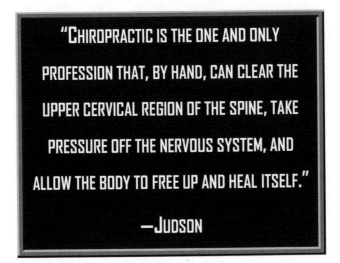

"CHIROPRACTIC IS THE ONE AND ONLY PROFESSION THAT, BY HAND, CAN CLEAR THE UPPER CERVICAL REGION OF THE SPINE, TAKE PRESSURE OFF THE NERVOUS SYSTEM, AND ALLOW THE BODY TO FREE UP AND HEAL ITSELF."

—JUDSON

Sperm meets egg. It's how life begins for us all. From that first moment, your cells immediately start dividing and multiplying. It is the beginning of a complicated and amazing process. It is the beginning of everything—the beginning of *you*.

One of the first things you developed as an embryo was a very tiny stalk: your spinal cord. At the top of that spinal cord, there was a little hump: your brain. The area where these two essential parts meet—the brain's connection to the spinal cord—is known as your brain stem.

You then developed a network of nerves branching out to every tissue of your growing body. Heart, liver, kidneys, lungs—everything. Those nerves were how your brain would communicate with your body throughout its development and for the rest of your life; it's how your body knows how to do *everything* it will ever need to do. And every one of those nerves begins its journey by leaving the brain and passing through the brain stem. When I was in school, they taught us that over 450 million nerve fibers traveled through the brain stem. That seemed like an awfully big number to me.

They were wrong. Now, we know that number is closer to 7 TRILLION.

As your body continued to grow in your mother's womb, your bones took form, beginning with a series of small bones encasing the spinal cord and brain stem: your vertebrae. Your vertebrae's job was (and is) to protect your spinal cord while also maintaining a necessary degree of flexibility.

Two specific vertebrae at the very top of the spine are devoted to protecting the brain stem: two small bones known as your **ATLAS** and your **AXIS**.

> **The ATLAS and the AXIS are the two most important bones in the human body, and most people have never even heard of them.**

Your vertebrae protect your spinal cord for a very important reason. As the location of your central nervous system, your spinal cord is the information superhighway upon which *every single message* between your brain and body is carried. If your spinal cord were to become damaged, those messages would be interrupted, resulting in a catastrophic loss of communication, leading to system-wide failure.

Do you remember Christopher Reeve, the actor who played Superman? His career was brought to a tragic end after a neck injury that caused complex fractures to his first and second cervical vertebrae (the atlas and the axis[1]). This devastating accident resulted in paralysis from the neck down—a complete and total disruption of communication between the nerves and the body. This is precisely

---

[1] Romano, Lois, "Riding Accident Paralyzes Actor Christopher Reeve," *The Washington Post*, June 1, 1995, A01.

why the brain stem is so important. It is also why the atlas and the axis are, hands down, the most important bones in your body.

The basic principle of chiropractic is that there are lesser degrees of spinal injuries not as immediate or as instantly severe as a total disruption of communication. These injuries are sometimes so small that they go unnoticed.

Vertebral Misalignments

Every vertebra is separated from its neighbors by soft discs of cartilage that act as ligaments holding your spine together. Your vertebrae float on these discs in order to provide flexibility to your spine. In other words, they can move. And as a result, they can sometimes slip out of their proper alignment.

Vertebral misalignments happen all the time and for a variety of reasons—taking a hard fall as a kid, getting "whiplash" from a fender bender, or just sleeping on your neck wrong. You might feel a misalignment when it happens, but then again you might not. The muscles around the area might feel sore at first, but muscles by their very nature are meant to adapt to resistance. (That's why weight training works to build muscle mass!) After a little time has passed, the muscles around the injured area will compensate for the new, incorrect position of the vertebrae. The soreness will lessen. Soon, you might be led to believe that whatever was wrong with your neck/back must have resolved itself and everything's fine . . . until the next tiny misalignment happens and things get much, much worse.

Have you ever seen an older person with a severe curve to their spine? You think that happened all at once? No way. That is what seventy or eighty years of cumulative vertebral misalignments looks like. You are seeing a lifetime of tiny, barely perceptible vertebral movements that have gone untreated.

A misalignment anywhere along the spine can put pressure on the spinal cord and affect the nervous system, but when it happens in the upper cervical area of your spine, the area of the atlas and the axis, that is when things get critical.

When the atlas and axis shift out of alignment, they can actually torque the brain stem itself, which puts direct pressure on your brain, disrupting the flow of messages to your central nervous system and affecting your body in a multitude of ways. This can cause issues as minor as localized pain or numbness in the extremities, or it can cause severe chemical imbalances, reduced organ function, and disease.

The critical question is, can this problem be corrected? Yes. And it's pretty simple. We find out exactly where there's a misalignment, and we gently move the vertebra back into its proper place. What I've just described is called a **CHIROPRACTIC ADJUSTMENT**.

The Chiropractic Adjustment and Living Clear

Since, as I mentioned, the muscles surrounding vertebrae naturally compensate for misalignments in the spine, it can take several chiropractic adjustments to get an adjustment to "hold." This is why chiropractors often tell their patients to come back next week.

Here's some friendly advice: Listen to your chiropractor's advice.

Even if you feel better after just one adjustment—even if your neck pain seems like it went away—go back for that next appointment. Trust me. Your chiropractor is not trying to get you to come back just to increase his or her business! We are doctors. We are charged with taking care of you, and we take that responsibility seriously; we're trying to get you to come back for your own good.

People who are under regular chiropractic care get checked consistently for misalignments. They are adjusted *only* when necessary and are examined regularly to determine how well and how long their bodies are holding an adjustment.

When your body can effectively hold an adjustment and you're getting checked for misalignments—correcting them *before* they become a problem—we call that LIVING CLEAR. That's when the upper cervical spine is clear of interference, and the nervous system is free of pressure.

When that happens, your body is able to heal itself.

The Fundamental Truths of Human Health

> ### Truth #1: HEALTH is your body's ability to perform.

Our modern concept of health care is heavily rooted in *treatment*. Not the treatment of people, unfortunately, but the treatment of disease. A better word for this model would be "sick-care."

In this multiple-diagnoses, multiple-prescriptions world, many of us have lost sight of what it means to be healthy, but it's not complicated. If you are performing at 100 percent of your body's potential, you are healthy, and there's absolutely no reason any symptom should present itself in your body. Most of us intuitively understand that, but we don't always think about it that way.

> ### Truth #2: When PERFORMANCE suffers, symptoms appear.

When the body's **PERFORMANCE** starts to reduce to lower than 100 percent, you start to notice that something is wrong. You don't feel right. Symptoms start to present themselves.

When symptoms get bad enough, you start looking for help. A medical doctor might even diagnose you with a disease or disorder, and you can't help but wonder where this problem came from. How did this happen?

> **Truth #3: When <u>SYMPTOMS</u> present themselves, it is the body's way of communicating an underlying problem.**

Let's turn back the clock. Did you *always* feel this way, or did it come about suddenly? Or was it a gradual process? Problems don't just spontaneously manifest within the body for no reason, yet that is often exactly how we think about health problems—they "just happen." *False!*

There is a cause and effect for everything that happens in your body. Whatever your symptoms are, **THERE IS A REASON** you feel the way you feel.

Let's follow the evidence. Let's track this problem down to see if we can figure out where it came from.

The Chiropractic Chemistry of Life

> **Your body's performance is controlled by your body's <u>CHEMISTRY</u>.**

In fact, your body is basically one big chemical reaction. Thousands of chemical reactions are going on inside you right now, helping your body adapt from the inside-out to any stressor you could throw at it. Every single biological function relies on this process.

If your performance is at less than 100 percent, it can be concluded that your body isn't adapting as optimally as it should, which means your body chemistry is at less than 100 percent.

Your body chemistry is controlled by your GLANDS.

Your glands are what produce all the chemicals used for all those reactions in your body. When your glands are operating at 100 percent, they can chemically react to your body's environment and help you adapt. But when they can't, that does not happen.

Commercials for prescription drugs constantly use the term "chemical imbalance" to explain health issues. All that really means is that when you have too much of one chemical in your body and not enough of another, things don't work the way they're supposed to.

Most prescription drugs work by artificially inducing your glands to produce more or less of a certain chemical. This artificial chemical balance is an attempt to return your body to its natural state of equilibrium, making you feel better (hopefully). But even when we do manage to regain that balance through artificial means, it still doesn't explain what is going on. We still aren't any closer to understanding *why* your glands are not working as intended. What caused your glands to behave his way in the first place?

I'll answer your question with another question: What controls your glands?

Your glands are controlled by your CENTRAL NERVOUS SYSTEM.

Your central nervous system doesn't just control your glands. It controls everything.

The nerves in your body serve two purposes.

1. Carrying messages *from the brain* to the body
2. Relaying information *to the brain* back from the body

Anytime you do something simple—for example, picking up a pencil—your body is responding to a message from your brain. You think it, your nerves relay the message, and your hand does what your brain tells it to do. When you feel the pencil between your fingers, that is function number two: your body sending sensory information back to your brain, and your brain decoding and interpreting the information.

Messages are being sent and received along the "power lines" of your central nervous system every instant of every day of your entire life. It isn't just about interacting with the outside world. Your brain is constantly sending messages to every part of your body. Telling your lungs to breathe. Telling your heart to beat. And telling your glands how to function.

> **If your glands are functioning at something less than 100 percent, we can conclude that your central nervous system is functioning at something less than 100 percent.**

How does the central nervous system work? What might affect it? What protects it from stress and interference so it can do its job?

> **The VERTEBRAE of the spine protect the central nervous system.**

The circular pieces of bone we call vertebrae act like armor. Their main function is to protect your spinal cord and your brain stem—the bottommost portion of your brain—which is housed within the top two vertebrae of your spine. I also mentioned in the previous section that your vertebrae float on discs of cartilage because your spine must maintain a certain degree of flexibility, meaning your vertebrae have the potential to rotate or tilt slightly out of proper alignment.

Sometimes, vertebrae move out of alignment and stay that way. This can result in back or neck pain. This is when most people come to see a chiropractor for the first time.

Back and neck pain are symptoms, and as we've learned, symptoms are simply manifestations of underlying problems—your body's warning system. Meanwhile, if a vertebra is misaligned enough to cause outward symptoms, what's going on *within* the spinal cord?

A piece of hard bone is pressing against your soft spinal cord. What's happening to that bundle of nerves it is meant to be protecting?

> It has been PROVEN that pressure on the spinal cord disrupts the function of nerves.

If a vertebra is out of alignment, it can put pressure on the spinal cord, kind of like a kink in a garden hose. Imagine if your atlas and/or axis are out of alignment. Now, it's not just your spinal cord feeling the pressure; it's your brain itself!

Have you ever wondered where your chronic headaches are coming from? Maybe it's stress. . . . Or maybe it's a piece of *hard bone* pushing against your soft brain!

If we follow the progression of how the body naturally functions, it always leads us back to the central nervous system, which always leads us to the spinal vertebrae. If a spinal vertebra slips out of alignment, it leads to. . . .

- Reduced *nervous system* function
- Reduced *gland* function
- Less than optimal body *chemistry*
- Less than 100 percent *performance*
- Symptoms

It all looks something like this.

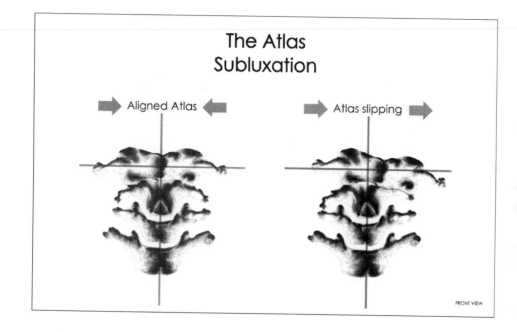

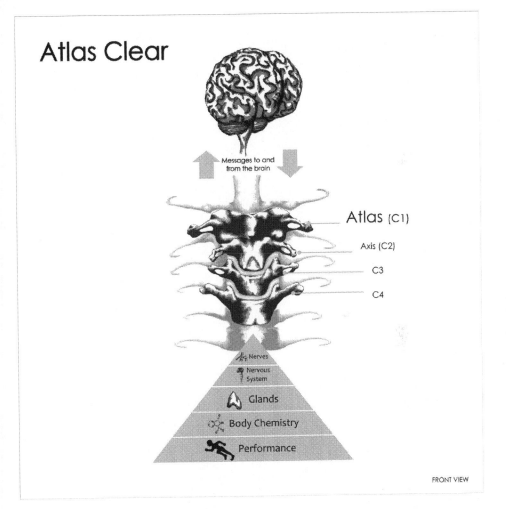

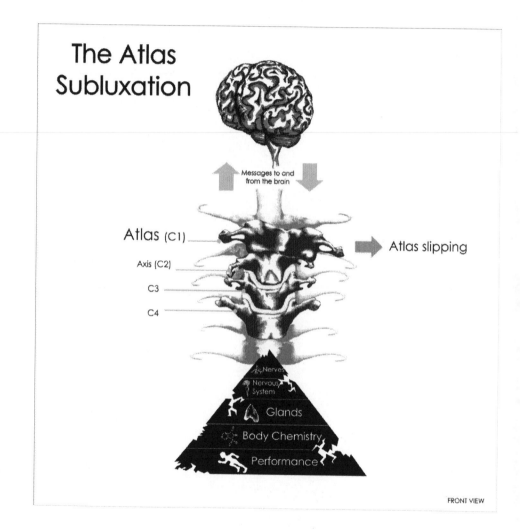

The Atlas Subluxation

Messages to and from the brain

Atlas (C1) — Atlas slipping

Axis (C2)

C3

C4

Nerves
Nervous System
Glands
Body Chemistry
Performance

It's basic math: If a misaligned upper cervical vertebra is disrupting nerve flow and allowing only 75 percent of your brain's vital messages to get through, then your body is performing 25 percent less efficiently than it should be. If only 50 percent of the messages are getting through, you're functioning at half your potential. And if you drop below 50 percent, things get really bad really fast.

The atlas and the axis—your first and second cervical vertebrae—are the most important elements in this equation because when your upper cervical spine is at less than 100 percent, it means the rest of you is at less than 100 percent by default.

What Do Chiropractors Do?

The job of the chiropractor has been miscommunicated thanks to years of unclear or flat-out inaccurate messages. People think our job is to relieve neck and/or back pain. Here's the truth:

> **The chiropractor's job is to take care of your central nervous system.**

Other than the brain itself, there's *nothing* more important than your central nervous system. If your digestive system starts shutting down, you get heartburn, stomach cramps, indigestion, things like that. If your circulatory system starts shutting down, you get numbness, tingling, fatigue, changes in body temperature, etc. But your nervous system controls *everything*. When that shuts down, everything else stops, too. You're dead. End of story.

In spite of all this, very few people realize the importance of nervous system health, which is kind of strange, when you think about it. And even though your vertebrae are the nervous system's only line of defense, hardly anybody talks about spinal health. In today's world, most people worry more about their colon than their brain stem. Hell, we learn more about taking care of our teeth as kids than we do about taking care of our nervous systems or our spines. But guess what: You can live without your teeth!

Most of us neglect the health of our nervous systems our entire lives, then wake up at forty or fifty years old and wonder why we're falling apart. But hey, at least our teeth look nice, right?

If I were to distil the information in this book down to a few key points, it would be as follows:

- **Your body is powerful from within.**
- **There is no chemical, physical, or emotional stress that your body cannot heal on its own.**
- **There is universal intelligence in all matter.**
- **Universal intelligence governs all matter and gives it all its properties and actions to maintain its existence.**
- **That intelligence flows through your central nervous system.**
- **Your nervous system travels from your brain to your body through your spine.**
- **The vertebrae in your spine sometimes become turned, tilted, or misaligned.**
- **When one or more vertebrae in your spine become misaligned, it can interfere with the function your nervous system.**

- When there is interference in your nervous system, less than 100 percent of the messages from your brain will reach your body.
- When your body receives less than 100 percent of your brain's messages, it cannot function as intended; it cannot heal itself.
- When you are clear of interference, 100 percent of your brain's messages reach your body.
- When your brain's messages reach your body, your body can heal.

If all you are interested in is treating symptoms, I guarantee modern medicine has a drug for it. There are pills to wake up, and pills to fall asleep. Pills to numb your headache—just to get it back again later. Pills to lose the weight—just to gain it back next week. Pills to lower your blood pressure—just to see it rise again. And, of course, pills to fix the side effects of all the pills you're taking.

The philosophy of chiropractic is to take care of the whole person, not just their symptoms. The mission is to restore the person to a state of normalcy so that the body can heal itself, reconnect, and function at a higher level.

The CHIROPRACTIC PRINCIPLE is about clearing out nervous system interference.
When your nervous system is clear, life is amazing.

When people are clear of nervous system interference, they can heal. This can manifest in extraordinary and sometimes unexpected ways. Whether it's chronic pain, seizures, migraines, or bedwetting—if you can name it, I've probably seen it. But being clear is about so much more than just being symptom-free. When you're clear, you can access your soul and determine, "What is my purpose on this earth?"

What are you doing with your life right now? What are you *supposed* to be doing? Are we supposed to just wake up every day, go to jobs we hate, come home, yell at our spouses, gorge ourselves at dinner, watch TV to forget about the stress for a while, go to bed angry, wake up depressed, and do it all over again? If that's our existence, what's the value in it?

What I'm trying to tell you is that the mission of the principled chiropractor is bigger than back pain. Chiropractic is about removing nervous system interference, letting the body take over, and giving people the chance to live the best life possible. It's about restoring health and ease to human beings so they can realize their dreams.

Chiropractic is about life, and *nothing* is bigger than life.

> *"Nothing is bigger than Life."*
> —*Dynamic Essentials mission statement*

What we need is to gain the clarity as a society about what the nervous system does. If more doctors could step up and educate their patients on taking care of the integrity of the nervous system—which essentially means seeing a principled chiropractor regularly—the entire world would change.

When you step foot in a principled chiropractor's office, you're deciding that you don't want to choose the path of least resistance and spend your whole life popping pills. By choosing to receive specific, scientific chiropractic care, you're attaining a next-level existence. You're choosing life instead of death.

Life is simply better with chiropractic.

What you have just read is essentially a "new patient orientation" at Judson Family Chiropractic. In my office, we are big on education. We always want to make sure you understand the process of chiropractic care—what we are doing, why we are doing it, how it works, and why it will help you. This is sometimes an uphill battle because chiropractic has become so misunderstood.

No one seems to understand what we really do! Heck, a lot of practicing chiropractors don't even seem to know, but I'll get to *them* later. . . .

Once and for all, let me clear up the confusion:

> **Chiropractic is THE ONE AND ONLY profession that, by hand, can clear the upper cervical region of the spine, take pressure off the nervous system, and allow the body to free up and heal itself.**

Honestly, there are really only a couple of techniques principled chiropractors use to clear out the brain stem. Other than the essential tools—our bare hands—we use only one or two other instruments to check a person to see if they're clear. We check the spine for misalignments. If we find one, we adjust it. That's it. That's all we do.

It's funny, but one of the arguments people make against chiropractic is that the same service we provide with our bare hands—taking pressure off the nervous system—can be done through high-tech surgical procedures conducted with precision tools. But before you hop on the operating table, I recommend you call up a surgeon and ask how invasive that kind of procedure will be. Ask if there are any potential risks involved in being put to sleep, opened up, hacked up inside, and stitched up again. Ask about recovery time, prescription painkillers, follow-up appointments, and possible complications or side effects.

How is that even comparable to having someone gently touch you with their bare hands?

My brother Ronnie lost his life because no one shared the truth of chiropractic with my family. The purpose of this book is to prevent that from happening to you or anyone you love. I intend to provide you with the knowledge you need to live clear, heal, and thrive.

As testimony to how chiropractic can change your life, let me share with you how it changed mine.

Chapter 2

My Story

I have been practicing chiropractic since 2002. My life has been a wild ride with a lot of bumps in the road, and I have only just recently started to think of myself as a grown-up. (The more gray hair I see, the harder it gets to ignore.) But I've always thought of myself as a blessed child. A blessed boy who became a blessed man.

As a kid growing up in New York with my mom, dad, brother, and sister, I was, to put it mildly, a total spaz. Yeah, I was *that* kid. I was always doing something crazy, always getting hurt. I busted my nose about three times before I even started playing sports.

As I got a little older, sports became my outlet, my passion, and my purpose in life. I think everybody at that age has a "superhero person" you look up to. For me, it was my big brother Ronnie.

Ronnie Judson wasn't just *my* hero. He was the guy all the kids in our town looked up to. He was a smaller guy, but he was tough, good-looking, ripped—just a stud. He worked out all the time and developed into an amazing athlete in high school in addition to being an A-plus student. He was a football star with a brilliant mind, and he became fluent in three languages. People loved him, and everyone knew he was going places.

Like many kids, I was a child of divorce and a brutal one at that, and Ronnie was the person I could always turn to. He was an amazing role model. The two of us shared a small bedroom and would have late-night talks when things got tough. It was the kind of cool brother stuff you never forget.

In some ways, Ronnie cast a big shadow. I remember going through school and all the teachers expecting big things from me because I was Ronnie's little brother. They expected me to be fluent in Spanish, too. Yeah, right! It didn't take long before I proved it didn't matter *whose* brother I was; I wasn't going to learn Spanish. I was not an A-plus student like Ronnie. I wasn't high honors. When my teachers noticed I wasn't doing so great in school, I was diagnosed with dyslexia. I don't know if ADD was a thing yet back then, but I probably would have been diagnosed with that, too.

There's one memory from elementary school that really stands out in my mind. It was when we were memorizing our "times tables." You know—two times one is two, two times two is four, two times three is six, so on and so forth. I remember we had a chart in our classroom with the times tables on it all the way up to twelve, with all the students' names written on it to record our progress. Each time you memorized one of your times tables, you got a little star beside your name. I will never forget looking up at that chart one day and realizing all the other kids had long rows of stars, and I only had two. I don't think I completely understood what that meant at the time, but I don't think I liked it.

That was just one of the many times when experiences in school made me feel like I was *not good enough*. The education system is a little different now, but back then, school really positioned kids like me for failure. The feelings of failure I began to experience led to some seriously toxic thoughts, even at a young age. Those toxic thoughts led to aggression, and sooner or later, one way or another, aggression always comes out.

The place where my aggression came out was on the athletic field, and after I started, there was no stopping me. I always went all-out and gave it everything I had. I sustained about seven diagnosed concussions as a result, but I became a really good athlete.

I had a lot of anger in me, probably because I had a lot to prove. After all, Ronnie Judson was my big brother. I felt like I had a lot to live up to, even though Ronnie never did or said anything to make me feel that way. Instead, Ronnie was the one who always lifted me up.

One of the coolest things in my young life was when I finally started coming into my own as a baseball player. It was around this time that my dream to be a professional pitcher took form. During one game in summer ball when I was a teenager, I was pitching with the game was on the line. It was the classic story: final inning, bases loaded, two outs, and it all came down to me. The place was packed. Everyone was watching. The pressure was intense. I hauled back, fired off my pitch, and struck the guy out for the final out and the win. My teammates started cheering. Ronnie wasn't even on the team, but he jumped the fence, came sprinting across the field to the mound, and picked me right up off the ground. I'll never forget that feeling. I was *someone* in that moment. I was a baseball player. I'd made my own little mark, and Ronnie was right there, literally lifting me up.

The Day Ronnie Judson's Life Was Stolen

After he graduated high school, Ronnie went off to college. I remember he wanted to go to West Point, but you know how it is. When you're the town star, everyone feels like they own a piece of you, as if you're somehow accountable to them for how you use your talent. Everybody told Ronnie he had to go to an Ivy League college and pursue sports because he was such a gifted athlete. So instead of West Point, he went to the University of Pennsylvania and pitched on the baseball team. He actually pitched a no-hitter against Yale, which I think is one of maybe only six in the school's history.

He went out for the football team, too. They made him a safety because they said he wasn't big enough to be a linebacker, but he was determined to prove them wrong. And he did. Through lots training and hard work, he won the starting linebacker spot for the UPenn football team. By all standards, Ronnie's life was pretty perfect. He was killing it on the athletic field while keeping his grade point average around the 3.6 or 3.7 mark. Everyone was proud of him, especially me.

Then one day, we got a phone call, and everything changed.

It took a while to learn the full story, but apparently, the football team had been doing some open-field tackling drills during an ordinary practice. These drills basically involve two guys lining up thirty or forty yards away, then running at each other. One guy is trying to get through; the other guy is trying to prevent it. The result is a tackle.

Usually, these drills are fairly routine. Other times, they can get downright ugly. Have you ever seen those videos of two bighorn sheep facing off and ramming their heads together? If things get out of hand, it can go something like that.

Like I said, Ronnie was a smaller guy. It had taken a lot of hard work for him to earn his position as linebacker in the first place, but he was tough. So when he got matched up against a 285-pound lineman, it didn't faze him.

I wasn't there that day, but what happened next replays itself in my mind almost every day of my life. Ronnie and the other guy lined up against one another across the open field. The coach blew the whistle. Ronnie went all-out, as he always did, and ran to meet the guy in a head-on collision. They smashed into one another, and Ronnie's neck snapped.

"I Don't Know What's Wrong with Me"

Ronnie woke up in the hospital.

My family and I arrived as quickly as we could, with everyone fearing the worst. After a bunch of X-rays, CT scans, and MRIs, the doctors told Ronnie he was very lucky. They said Ronnie's neck had twisted so badly that he had been millimeters away from being either killed or paralyzed from the neck down. The rest of the news was no surprise: Ronnie could never play football—or any other sports—ever again. But the important part was he had dodged a bullet. He was going to be okay.

And that was it. In a split second, Ronnie's athletic career was over, but at least he was alive. The doctors gave him three prescription medications and sent him back to school in a neck brace.

The collective response from family and friends was, "Phew! Thank God! That was a close one." Everyone was sad he had lost his chance to be a star athlete, but that didn't matter. He was going to be okay. He was still a smart, hard-working guy getting a great education at a top university. One option was off the table, but he still had everything going for him.

That was what we all thought, anyway. None of us knew it at the time, but that event marked the beginning of the end of Ronnie's life.

***

My big brother had been a healthy, intelligent, motivated guy everyone wanted to be around. But all that changed after his injury.

Suddenly, Ronnie was sick all the time. This was not normal for him. He had always been fit and healthy. It got so bad that the doctors took out his tonsils because they thought it might help with his recurring sicknesses, but it did nothing.

Then Ronnie's grades started slipping. For the first time in his life, he was having trouble in school. Again, this was not normal for him. Soon, he confided to me that he was having strange, dark thoughts. He couldn't sleep, so he started going out late at night. He couldn't concentrate—couldn't focus on his schoolwork—and his grades went from slipping to plummeting. He suffered from depression and anxiety. He started drinking and partying to try to calm down his system and quiet those strange thoughts, and it was not long before he started getting into trouble.

One night, about six months after Ronnie got out of the hospital, I was sitting at dinner with my mother when the doorbell rang. I will never forget it. I opened the front door to find Ronnie just standing there. At least, it *looked* like Ronnie. But I swear, when I opened that door, I was looking into the eyes of a different human being.

This was not the Ronnie Judson I knew. This was not my brother.

Ronnie walked into the house. He looked at me with this haunted expression on his face and said, "I need help, Steve. . . . I don't know what's wrong with me."

My parents took Ronnie to one of the top psychiatrists in the area. The specialists there suspected that something had just "snapped" in him mentally, so they ran a bunch of tests to try to figure out what it was and how to treat it. They did an intensive psychiatric review, a five-hour-long analysis.

At the end of the analysis, the head psychiatrist came out and sat down with my parents. "There's nothing wrong with this kid," he said. "Don't let him ruin an Ivy League education. Get him back in school."

So, trusting the doctors' professional opinions, my parents put Ronnie on a train and sent him back to UPenn. It seemed like the right thing to do.

Within hours, we got a call from the Philadelphia Police Department. Ronnie had gotten off his train, walked right up to some random gang in South Philly, and challenged them all to a fight.

Ask anyone who knows, and they will tell you that what Ronnie did that night was as good as committing suicide. No one does something like that unless they have a death wish. These guys could have killed Ronnie right there—beaten him down and buried him in the street. On any other night, who knows? Maybe they would have. But instead, for whatever reason, the head of this gang told his buddies, "Leave this guy alone," and *they* called the police to report that there was some crazy guy roaming the streets trying to get himself killed. The cops came and picked Ronnie up.

That little stunt landed Ronnie in a psychiatric hospital. It would be the first of many.

What the Heck is a Chiropractor?

As for me, I was still in high school and doing my best to follow in my brother's footsteps. Like I said, I got hurt a lot. I had seven concussions, broke my nose a bunch of times, and probably cracked every rib in my body. I suffered from migraines every single day, carried a lot of pain in my lower back, and averaged about three hours of sleep a night.

I was a pretty good pitcher, but it was around this time that I tore my rotator cuff. It's a very common injury among pitchers and has ended many a young man's athletic career. Overnight, all my dreams of becoming a major league pitcher vanished into thin air.

Sports were supposed to be my thing. That was what I did!

Now what?

By the end of my junior year of high school, my mom was working for a chiropractor. She started telling me, "*You're* going to be a chiropractor, Steve."

I said, "What the heck is that?"

She punched me in the chest and repeated, "You're going to be a chiropractor, Steve."

For years, she did that. She would punch me in the chest and say those words. She was a little Irish lady, but she wore this big, gold ring, so you really felt those hits. It's funny, because I've since learned about neurolinguistic programming, and that's exactly what she was doing, whether she realized it or not. Every time she punched me in the chest and said, "You're going to be a chiropractor, Steve," it planted a seed in me, forming a connection in my brain and becoming part of my subconscious. I would never forget her words . . . or the impact of that gold ring.

This Is Life Now

Over time, my migraines got worse and worse. Nothing seemed to help. Pretty much by accident, I ended up in a chiropractor's office and received my first chiropractic adjustment. (Of course, I now know it was no accident.)

This chiropractor adjusted me, and I came back about five times after that. The pain in my lower back got a lot better, and my migraines went away. The problem was, there was no carryover. The guy didn't educate me on anything he was doing or why he was doing it, so when I started feeling better, I stopped going. I never spoke to him again.

This scenario is typical of many people's experiences with a chiropractor—effective but short-lived. It wouldn't be until years later that I thought back to that first adjustment and my mom's words and said, "You know what? That was kind of cool. I gotta find out more about that chiropractic stuff." But more on that later.

Meanwhile, my brother was not getting any better. His depression and anxiety were getting progressively worse, and he was eventually diagnosed with multiple mental disorders including schizophrenia and bipolar disorder. He was constantly in and out of psychiatric institutions for treatment.

The most frustrating part was that it made no sense! Why was this happening to him? Where did these problems come from? Why would multiple mental disorders manifest so suddenly in an otherwise healthy, young guy? Whenever my parents would ask the doctors about it, their answer was, "These things just happen sometimes."

The doctors told us how mental disorders can manifest in adolescence and present themselves years later. Other doctors would say things like, "Well, maybe the stress just finally got to him." It sounded like a guess! They had no idea how to fix this thing. All they did was treat his symptoms. Their message was pretty much, *This is his life now, and you'll just have to learn to cope with it.*

On the weekends, I would drive out with my girlfriend to visit Ronnie at whatever hospital he was in at the time, which could sometimes be a pretty horrifying experience. The things I saw in those institutions were disturbing.

One patient had been a big-shot lawyer. Another had been a successful accountant, though you wouldn't have known it to look at them. It was surreal and a little scary to see these people who had once been normal, now reduced to this. They were no longer able to even function outside a hospital. I would hear their stories, and all I could do was shake my head and say, "Poor guy. . . ." Luckily, Ron didn't seem to have it as bad as they did. Things were rough, sure, but his problems didn't seem so bad by comparison. He was actually dating one of the nurses at one point! It was pretty wild.

It was scary to see the people who were *really* bad. They were alive and walking around, but it was like the lights were out. You could look into their eyes, and it was like life had left the body. I found myself wondering, what the heck happened to them to make them this way? Did all this stuff lay dormant in them and manifest all of a sudden, like the doctors said had happened to Ronnie? If they *used* to be okay, what was different now? They had been normal at some point, right? So what changed?

But what really hit me hard was when I realized some of these people's stories were hauntingly similar to Ronnie's.

In fact, there were people in these institutions who had been through *the same thing* as my brother. These had lived their entire lives without any diagnosis. Then they sustained an injury—sometimes sports-related, sometimes a car or motorcycle accident, or sometimes just a bad fall—and suddenly developed a psychological disorder. Was it all just coincidence?

Despite this common theme, there was really never any discussion about head or neck injuries. The doctors in these places weren't there to determine the *cause* of their patients' difficulties; their job was to *treat* these people's symptoms. And treating symptoms, I started to realize, meant giving drugs. Lots of drugs.

***

After I graduated high school, I went off to college. I had no idea what I wanted to do with my life. At one point, I wanted to be a lawyer. Then I saw my buddy studying for his law exams, and I was like, "*I'm* not doing all that freaking reading." Then I got the idea that I was going to be a motivational speaker. I was all over the place. I ultimately majored in English. Why English? Because despite having no passion for it, I could write a fifty-page paper in a night. I had never been a good student, so I figured I might as well choose a major that came easily to me.

It was true that I wasn't the sharpest tool in the shed, but the problem wasn't my intelligence. It was that I just didn't give a crap. My brother's story had made me bitter, and I pretty much thought school was a bunch of bullshit. I didn't know what I was doing or where I was going. I would slog through my classes, then go home to a broken family—divorced parents, a brother in a psychiatric hospital, and a sister it was up to me to take care of. There were days when I didn't even want to be alive because of the amount of pain I felt.

I visited Ronnie every chance I got. Like I said, he had never been as bad off as the other patients in those places . . . but gradually, I saw that start to change.

Ronnie's health was declining. He started to look worse and worse over time. He was changing—and not just physically. He would sometimes say or do things that were totally out of character. The medications, I realized, were changing him, and it was a frightening thing to watch.

At first, his friends had been there for him. That changed, too. For me, one of the hardest parts of watching his decline was seeing all his old buddies start to abandon him. They stopped visiting. They walked away and acted like he didn't exist anymore. I think part of it was fear of what had happened to him. He had gone from being this amazing person with a great life—the hometown hero, tons of friends, a bright future, everything going for him—to some guy stuck in a mental hospital, all alone. It got to the point where I almost wanted to fake a problem of my own and commit myself just to be by his side, to try to help him, to try to stop the madness.

My college experience rolled on. I had to work as a bartender and bouncer to make ends meet, so I was up until four or five in the morning most nights. Some days, I would literally go from the bar to breakfast to class. The best I can say is I was getting by.

One day, I told myself, "This isn't working, and you know it. English is not where you're meant to be." I still had no idea where I *was* meant to be, but at least I could rule that one out.

I went to my guidance counselor, and for some reason, in that moment as I sat down in his office, I thought back to the guy years before who had adjusted my neck and relieved my migraines. I thought back to my little, Irish mom and her gold ring punching me in the chest. *You're going to be a chiropractor, Steve.*

I asked the guidance counselor, "What does it take to be a chiropractor?"

"Not you," he said.

I said, "Why?"

He pulled out my folder and my career development testing and looked it over. Everything about my scores screamed management, public speaking, or an English-related field. As far as *science*, the graphs were literally going in the opposite direction. Like I said, English came easy. Science and math, not so much.

"See?" he said. "You're not cut out for it. You would fail."

I think he thought I was messing with him because at that point, he threw the folder at my chest and said, "Get out of my office. You're wasting my time."

I left thinking, *I'll prove you wrong, pal.*

I went to the registrar and enrolled in all the premed classes for chiropractic school. Maybe Mom had been right all along.

Chapter 3

Dynamic Essentials: My Call to Chiropractic

Now that I was officially enrolled in pre-med courses and chiropractic was in my sights, I got it into my head that I would be a sports chiropractor. I would work with professional athletes. I pictured myself running a big sports facility with a track outside where MLB and NFL stars would rehab and run. I was dreaming big, and I was motivated, no doubt about it. There was just one problem. . . .

I was failing *everything*.

I often tell people that I was just about the worst college student on Earth. My first semester in pre-med was evidence of that. It was a disaster. My grades were garbage. I got something like a 30 percent on my first midterm, and things did not get much better from there.

Finals came around. I failed Physics. I failed Biology. And after it was all over, I went out to the corner pub and had about twenty Guinnesses. I was just sitting there feeling sorry for myself when the words suddenly entered my head: *You didn't work hard enough.* I'm not sure where those words came from. Maybe from God. But I realized in that moment, "Wow. I really didn't."

As an English major, I had been able to coast along without trying very hard. I partied whenever I felt like it, and I definitely did not study as much as I should have. But this was not English. This was not something I was naturally good at. It was a whole new frontier, and I couldn't expect to succeed if I kept up the same old habits. I had to behave like an athlete and train and work hard every day to make it happen. Once I realized this, I was absolutely convicted of that truth. I re-enrolled. This time, I got tutors, and all I did was study. I didn't party. Every day, I would hole up in my room and listen to Van

Morrison's album *Moondance* while I studied. I would review what we had done the day before, then go back through all the notes, five hours a day, with Van Morrison on.

I saw myself as an underdog. I was a fighter getting in shape for a shot at the title. I had to *train* and be *disciplined* to do this.

I wish I could say my devotion to the process was because I felt called to a mission, but at that point, it was more about proving everyone else wrong and proving to myself that I could do this. There was no big "why" in my story yet.

Little did I know it was just around the corner.

***

After I finished my undergrad studies (by the skin of my teeth), I enrolled at Life University in Marietta, Georgia, which was just about the greatest chiropractic school in the world at the time. Life had been founded by Dr. Sid Williams, one of the most brilliant chiropractic educators and speakers who ever lived. He was the "mother lode of all chiropractors," and when I started at Life, he was the university's president. Dr. Sid also happened to be the first person I ran into on campus, and in the following years, he would become a mentor, a source of inspiration, and a close friend.

Of course, I didn't know any of this at the time.

Looking back on it now, it's almost funny. I ended up at Life because I was looking at different schools and thought, "You know what? I want to go somewhere warm. Oh, there's a school in Georgia? It's pretty warm there, right? Probably a good fit. Okay, I'll go there." I thought Life was just some chiropractic school, I was just some student who happened to go there, and Dr. Sid was just some teacher, right?

I hadn't been at Life very long when this goofy-looking guy with a ponytail came up to me on campus and said, "Hey, are you going to DE?"

I said, "DE?"

"It's a chiropractic seminar," he said. "Dynamic Essentials. You need to go!"

I asked him when it was, and he told me the date: ten weeks away. I said, "Okay, sure," and pretty much immediately forgot about it. After all, I was in chiropractic school for one reason: I wanted to adjust people! I wanted to get out into the world, start my business, start adjusting, and open up that big sports injuries facility I dreamed of.

That attitude ruled over my studies, too. I felt that all I needed to know was how to adjust. I didn't see the point of learning anatomy, physiology, or any of that stuff. I had beaten the odds just by making it here; *staying* here was my priority. I spent my whole first quarter working my butt off, studying hard, putting in the work, just trying to make it, really. I didn't see the point of going to seminars. Sitting through *more* lectures? Doing *extra* work? No thank you.

The Dynamic Essentials of Health

Chiropractic school was tough, but if there was one thing I had going for me, it was passion. Before I knew it, I'd made it through my first quarter. I didn't know how well I'd done on my finals, but at least they were *over*! I was ready to unwind, baby. My buddies were, too. We all planned to go to this huge party the night after finals, and man, was I ready!

I was walking across campus on my way home to get ready for the big party when I turned the corner and ran into an upperclassman. It was the kid with the ponytail from ten weeks earlier.

"Hey!" he said. "You going to DE?"

"Huh?" I said. "Oh, right. That seminar thing. When is it?"

He said, "It starts tonight."

"Oh," I said. "Well, maybe. . . ."

I said goodbye to the kid and went on my way. Tonight? Are you kidding me? The night after finals? No way! I was *partying* tonight!

Still, I had this strange feeling I should go.

I can't explain it. Somehow, it felt like I needed to be there for some reason. I figured, what could it hurt to stop in and see what it's all about? Maybe my buddies would want to go too, and then we could all head over the party. I got in touch with all my friends and tried to convince them to come with me.

"A *seminar*?" they said. "Classes are finally over, and now you wanna go sit through *another one*? Nah, no way man. School's out. Time to party."

"Yeah, okay," I said. "I'll see you soon."

They were right—this was no time for sitting through more lessons. I had worked hard all semester. Now was the time to unwind and celebrate.

I went home and showered, but that feeling was still there. I decided if my buddies didn't want to go, I would just drop by this Dynamic Essentials thing for myself, just for a couple of minutes. There would still be plenty of time to party. We had all night. What was a couple minutes just to check it out?

***

I walked into the auditorium where this chiropractic "seminar" was being held, and I was stunned.

I had been picturing a lecture. A classroom with students and some boring teacher at the front. But this was more like a rock concert. The place was packed. There must have been 1,500, maybe 2,000 people in there. Some of them were hugging each other, laughing, hollering— they were fired up!

What a bunch of freaks! I thought. *What the hell am I doing here? I ought to just walk out now.*

A few speakers got up onstage and started talking about chiropractic, but I wasn't really listening. I was just leaning against the wall in the back of the room, thinking, *Why am I even here? Why don't I just leave?*

I did actually leave. Or I tried to, anyway.

In fact, over the course of the next half-hour or so, I left five separate times, but every time I walked out, something pulled me back. Each time I tried to leave, I ended up in the bathroom where I would wash my face, then go back into the auditorium. I kept returning and leaning against that spot along the back wall.

Finally, this guy in a red blazer gets up onstage. The room goes silent. He introduces himself as Dr. Michael Kale, and he starts talking in this thick southern accent about the history of chiropractic, about Dr. D.D. Palmer, Dr. B.J. Palmer, and a place called the Clear View Sanitarium.

My life would never be the same again.

The History of Chiropractic

> *"Chiropractic is a philosophy, science and art of things natural; a system of adjusting the segments of the spinal column by hand only, for the correction of the cause of dis-ease."* [2]
>
> —B.J. Palmer

---

[2] Stephenson, Ralph W., *Chiropractic Textbook* (Davenport: The Palmer School of Chiropractic, 1948), xiii.

> *"Although Chiropractic was not so named until
> 1896 ... [it] dates back at least five years
> previous to 1895. During those five years, as I
> review many of these writings, I find they talk
> about various phases of that which now
> constitutes some of the phases of our present day
> philosophy, showing that my father was
> thinking along and towards those lines which
> eventually, suddenly crystallized in the
> accidental case of Harvey Lillard, after which it
> sprung suddenly into fire and produced the
> white hot blaze."[3]*
>
> —B.J. Palmer

That night, at Dynamic Essentials, I learned that the very first documented chiropractic patient was a man who had been deaf for seventeen years.

Three days after his first adjustment—the first chiropractic adjustment in history—the man could hear.

The year was 1895. Working out of an office in Davenport Iowa, Dr. Daniel David Palmer was researching the concept of healing without drugs, and believe me, this was just as radical a theory back then as it is today. On September 18, Harvey Lillard, the hearing impaired African-American janitor who worked on the building's fourth floor, entered D.D. Palmer's office complaining about neck pain. Out of curiosity, D.D. asked Lillard how he had lost his hearing. Lillard told him it had all started one day when he had simply bent down to pick up a box.

---

[3] Palmer, B.J. cited by Stephenson, *Chiropractic Textbook*, 230.

49

"While in a cramped, stooped position," Lillard said, "I felt and heard something pop in my back. Immediately, I went deaf."[4]

Dr. Palmer was, understandably, a little confused by Lillard's story. Why would a "pop" in your back have anything to do with your hearing? There was nothing in traditional medicine to suggest a functional connection between a person's back and their ears. Maybe it was just a coincidence. He asked to examine Lillard's back, and, to his surprise, easily located a strange *bump* in Lillard's spine. D.D.'s son B.J. Palmer later wrote:

> *"The patient was put upon the floor, face down, and a shove-like movement given. The 'bump' was reduced by the first three shoves, and in three days hearing was restored. Harvey could hear a watch tick at the average distance you and I can today."[5]*

The restoration of Harvey Lillard's hearing was clearly amazing, but it posed many questions. Why would someone's *spine* affect their *ears*? And why would reducing a *bump* restore a deaf man's hearing? If a bump in a certain area of the spine could cause deafness, then what could other bumps do, in other areas of the back? Did other people have similar bumps that were affecting their health? What other disorders, conditions, or diseases might these bumps be causing?

Could health problems actually be eased, or even healed, by correcting problems in the spine?

Today, D.D. Palmer's adjustment of Harvey Lillard's spine is considered the birth of the chiropractic profession, and the "bump" was the first observed vertebral subluxation.

---

4 Stephenson, *Chiropractic Textbook*, 231.
5 Palmer, B.J. cited by Stephenson, *Chiropractic Textbook*, 231.

The Vertebral Subluxation: The Root of Human Disease

> *"If the reduction of one bump in one man restores hearing, why won't a similar bump in other people, produce deafness, and if it does, why wouldn't the reduction of these bumps in the same way, restore their hearing? . . . If a bump in the back caused deafness, why not other parts of the spine produce other dis-ease?"*
>
> —B.J. Palmer

There had been spinal adjusters before D.D. Palmer, but it took that perfect set of circumstances on that September day in Iowa to bring the full reality of chiropractic to light.

Dr. Palmer's second patient was a woman with heart issues who, as it turned out, also had a bump in her spine similar to the one discovered on Lillard. Dr. Palmer decided to try to help her by using the same technique. Sources say the results didn't come quite as readily as they had with Lillard, but the woman's heart problems got increasingly better as the bump in her spine was reduced.

At this point, D.D. Palmer did not know *why* adjusting the spine helped people heal, but he did know there was no way it was a coincidence! If a spinal adjustment could affect the ears *and* the heart, then there must have been something going on in the human spine that no one had ever fully understood before. He named this new process **CHIROPRACTIC.** (Most people are surprised to learn that the word *chiropractic* has nothing to do with the spine or the back. It means "done by hand.")

D.D. concluded that if the spine was the source of so much disease—or *dis-ease*, as he preferred to call it—then it was important to know as much about the spine as possible. In the following years, he devoted himself to studying the spine, the vertebrae, the spinal nerves, and those strange bumps he kept finding. He examined patients and dissected cadavers and painstakingly diagrammed the spinal nerves. He soon learned that the strange bumps he kept finding were actually misaligned vertebrae. He theorized that the normal function of spinal nerves was being *interrupted* by these misalignments. When vertebrae became misaligned, or "subluxated," as he called it, it impinged the spinal nerves, interrupting the flow of impulses and signals to the rest of the body, resulting in an interruption of the body's natural state of ease, thus producing "dis-ease."

> **SUBLUXATION**: The prefix **sub** means "less than" or "below." **Luxation** is another word for "dislocation." A subluxation is simply an injury that is less severe than a dislocation.

On the basis of D.D.'s theories, the fundamental idea behind chiropractic became as follows:

- The mechanics of the spine normally work perfectly, but their function can be interrupted by a **SUBLUXATION**

- Subluxations can put pressure on the whole system, disrupting the mechanics of the body

- Those same mechanics can also be *restored* if misaligned vertebrae are returned to their natural position, by hand, through a **CHIROPRACTIC ADJUSTMENT**

It was a huge breakthrough, but this was only the beginning.

Dr. B.J. Palmer's Law of Life

When Dr. D.D. Palmer died in 1913, his son B.J. Palmer picked up his father's legacy. Today, Dr. B.J. Palmer is known as the developer of chiropractic, and many of his studies are still considered some of the most authoritative research ever done on the function of the human spine and the nervous system as a whole. He expanded the field of chiropractic. The culmination was his "Law of Life."

Palmer's Law of Life

- There is a gigantic, exhaustless and intelligent power house resident in living man's brain.
- This intelligent power is sufficient unto man's every need if it gets from where it is to where it is needed.
- Sickness or dis-ease can exist anywhere, in any organ, in any manner, when this free flow power is interfered with between brain and body.
- What interferes, blocks, obstructs this unlimited supply?
- A twisted, distorted, abnormally positioned vertebra of the backbone, producing pressure upon the power-transmitting cord of nerves.
- This "shorts" the circuit downward from brain to body, and upward sense from body to brain.
- This condition causes every dis-ease, in every organ, in any form. What is necessary to be done to get sick people well?
- Correct, by hand only, the mal-positioned vertebral subluxation.
- Release pressures upon nerves.

- Permit a restoration of the imprisoned power supply from above-down, inside-out.
- Let it have free flow, normally.
- When it reaches dis-ease, ease follows of its own accord. This condition, from above-down, inside-out, cures every and all dis-ease. That is Palmer's simple and single Law of Life. A chiropractor, who knows chiropractic, who knows the Palmer Law of Life, knows how and does but one thing.
- Adjust the vertebral subluxation. . . .
- Letting intellectual power from above-downward, inside-out do the curing.

Soon, chiropractic was growing exponentially. In 1935, B.J. Palmer opened the Dr. B.J. Palmer Chiropractic Research Clinic in Davenport, Iowa. He later took over Clear View Sanitarium, a chiropractic psychiatric hospital. He spent his time researching a new chiropractic procedure focused specifically on the upper cervical region.

The stories about Clear View and B.J. Palmer's clinic are incredible. These days, every patient who enters my office receives a copy of an article written by L. Ted Frigard, a chiropractor who worked at B.J. Palmer's clinic in the 1950s. The article is an account of what happened when Dr. Charles Mayo, cofounder of the Mayo Clinic, brought his wife to see Dr. Palmer.[6] She was suffering from some health problems, and all attempts at medical treatment had failed to help her.

At Dr. Palmer's clinic, Mrs. Mayo began receiving upper cervical chiropractic adjustments. Dr. Mayo, who was not a believer in

---

[6] Frigard, L. Ted, "Dr. Palmer vs. Dr. Mayo," *Dynamic Chiropractic*, June 12, 2000, Vol. 18, Issue 13.

chiropractic whatsoever, questioned Dr. Palmer's methods and fought him every step of the way. In response, B.J. reportedly told him, "Dr. Mayo, while you are here, we are going to ask you to keep your mouth shut."[7]

Frigard goes on to state: "Mrs. Mayo received chiropractic care for several months and went home well. Dr. Mayo stated it was impossible for her to get well with what Palmer did, yet he also admitted she was well.... I was on the staff of the B.J. Palmer Chiropractic Clinic in 1953–54. Although 'Dr. Charlie' had passed away in 1939, during that time, 60 to 80 percent of our patients were referred by 'someone' on the staff of the Mayo Clinic."[8]

People came from around the country—around the world—to be helped by Dr. Palmer. It's said that his waiting room could hold hundreds of people and it was common for every seat to be filled. He and his team specialized in helping patients suffering from psychiatric and psychological problems by adjusting their upper cervical spines. And it worked.

Remember, we're not talking about some time in the distant past. It was the 1950s—well into the modern era, and well-documented by many sources. It was at a time when the medical community treated psychiatric and psychological disorders through the use of powerful drugs and other more questionable methods (the lobotomy comes to mind). If you couldn't be helped, you were removed from society, sedated, and confined to an asylum for the rest of your life. Plus, they might even drill a hole in your head, just for good measure.

Those were the stakes back then. If they couldn't cure you, you were sedated and locked away until you died.

The numbers indicate that 85 percent of patients at Clear View Sanitarium got well and were able to return to their normal lives thanks to upper cervical chiropractic adjustments, done by hand only.

---

7 Frigard, "Dr. Palmer vs. Dr. Mayo"
8 Frigard, "Dr. Palmer vs. Dr. Mayo"

Take a second to think about how amazing that truly is. These were people the medical community basically considered beyond hope. They were lost causes. They were people who would have otherwise been locked in a room, forever. And at Clear View, 85 percent of them were getting well. The symptoms of mental illnesses and psychiatric disorders weren't just being managed; they were being *reversed*.

These people were being healed.

***

So there I was, leaning against the back wall of the auditorium at this thing called Dynamic Essentials, listening to Dr. Kale and hearing all this for the first time in my life. I found myself hanging on his every word.

I was floored—I couldn't believe what he was saying! I thought chiropractic was just about relieving lower back pain, helping recover from injuries, increasing range of motion, and that sort of thing. But Dr. Kale was talking about people being healed of psychological disorders with upper cervical adjustments as far back as the *1930s*!

This upper cervical stuff was a form of chiropractic I had never been exposed to before, and it sounded nothing short of amazing. Dr. Kale went on to talk about how he was currently using the same kind of upper cervical adjustments to successfully help patients with psychological disorders in his office. He started describing some of the kinds of patients he was currently working with: people who had been in accidents that involved the upper cervical region that had put pressure on the brain stem. . . .

And suddenly, I started getting goosebumps. The reality hit me like a bomb. He was describing my brother.

He was telling Ronnie Judson's story.

I couldn't move. I could hardly breathe. Standing there, in that room of almost 2,000 people, it was like I was the only person on Earth—he was talking directly to me, telling me Ronnie's story—telling me *my* story!

I started to cry. *All* Ronnie's problems and disorders and diagnoses had begun the day he got hit. Everything could be traced back to his neck injury. I found myself flashing back to the doctors telling us that Ronnie's injury had compressed his brain stem. Since then, he had been treated like he was beyond hope, like he was a lost cause. . . .

But was he? Maybe there was an answer.

Maybe Ronnie could get help.

I stood pinned against that wall, paralyzed, weeping like a child, realizing that everything I had ever been through had been leading me here to this moment: the moment my whole life story came together. This was why I had needed to be here tonight. This was why something had stopped me five separate times from leaving the building. And this was why my journey had led me to chiropractic. It was the mission I had been plucked out of this world to fulfill.

This was why God chose me to do this.

When Dr. Kale walked off the stage, he went out into the room and started adjusting people. I left the back wall, went to the front of the room, and waited for my turn to be adjusted. It was a different kind of adjustment than I'd ever received before—a specialized kind that addressed the upper cervical region he had been talking about. I went home and went to sleep, and when I woke up, it felt like a vase had been lifted off my head. I realized I had been sleeping for eighteen hours straight. There was a sense of clarity I had never felt before. A sense of fulfillment. It was like waking up from a dream. That was when I knew I was on a mission. I needed to learn this. I was going to be a master at this, and I was going to bring it to the world.

That day, everything changed. I was pulled out of the cell of pain and heartache I'd been living in for all those years, brought to DE as a first-quarter student, and given the answer.

Chapter 4

A Deeper Look at Chiropractic

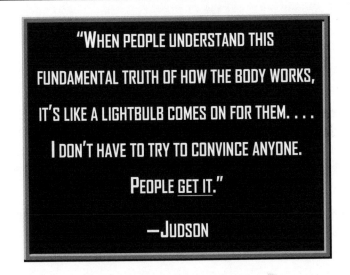

"WHEN PEOPLE UNDERSTAND THIS FUNDAMENTAL TRUTH OF HOW THE BODY WORKS, IT'S LIKE A LIGHTBULB COMES ON FOR THEM. . . . I DON'T HAVE TO TRY TO CONVINCE ANYONE. PEOPLE GET IT."

—JUDSON

Until that moment, my life had been in disarray. I hadn't known it at the time, but I had been walking around subluxated.

Sure, I had been adjusted before, but when Dr. Kale adjusted me at DE, that was my first *real* adjustment. After that, things changed for me in major ways. For the first time in my life, I knew what it meant to be **CLEAR**. It manifested in my health, my attitude, my grades—in just about every aspect of who I was. For the rest of my time in school, all I did was research, read, and study. I didn't party. From then on, I was acting according to my purpose, and I wasn't messing around anymore.

As it turned out, I was destined to be a pretty good student. Who knew? Funny story: When I finally realized *how* to be a good student, all it boiled down to was listening for little hints, like the spot in the lecture when the teacher subtly raised his voice. When I heard it, I thought, "Well, that question's gonna be on the test, probably." I was usually right. I'm sure this comes naturally for some people, but, like I said, I was one of those "spaz" kids growing up. For me, it was like, why couldn't I have figured this out twelve years ago?

Throughout my time at Life University, Dr. Sid Williams became a huge influence. Dr. Sid was a man of vision. All you had to do was shake his hand to feel the power he had. In 1974, he had founded Life Chiropractic College (later Life University), and he was serving as Life's president while I was attending. People called him the "Defender of Chiropractic" because he was directly responsible for saving our profession. In the dark years when chiropractic was falling apart (which I'll discuss in Chapter Eight), he was the one who stood in the center of that fire and never backed down. He was also the driving force behind Dynamic Essentials, the event that changed my life.

Anywhere Dr. Sid went to speak, I went and listened. I watched his videos. I read his books (and to this day, one book I am constantly recommending to young chiropractors, students, and humans in general is Dr. Sid's *The Meadowlands Experience*).

Eventually, I started just showing up at Dr. Sid's office on Life campus and talking to him one-on-one. The things he taught me about life, vision, loving people, serving people, transforming lives—I had never heard these things before, and those lessons played a major role in my development as a chiropractor and as a man.

The Nervous System

"Everything has a sufficient cause for being what it is—our health, our success and our place in the world in which we live. All of us have a

> *laboratory for conducting our scientific*
> *experiments. . . . If we are not satisfied with*
> *what we find, we take steps to improve our*
> *situation by the elimination of those things*
> *which are responsible and by substituting those*
> *things which would make our lives more*
> *satisfying."*[9]
>
> —*Carl Holmes*

The reason I started this book with a summary of the chiropractic chemistry of life instead of jumping straight into my personal story is because when people understand this fundamental truth of how the body works, it's like a lightbulb comes on for them. I see it all the time in my office. During education sessions and new patient orientations, all I have to do is pull back the veil and reveal this truth. I don't have to try to convince anyone. People *get it.*

Now that you know the basics of how the body performs and functions, it's time to take a more in-depth look at the human nervous system. You've had the milk. Now you're ready for the meat.

Within the human nervous system are trillions of individual nerves, all of which are comprised of axons—tiny filaments or branches—that travel throughout your body. Messages travel along this branching network in the form tiny electrical impulses. The ones that carry messages to the body—like the message your brain sends to your fingers when you decide to turn the page of a book—are called *efferent nerves.* Nerves that carry information back to the brain—like the sensation of pain if you get a paper cut—are *afferent nerves.*

Think of your efferent and afferent nerves like power lines running through your body. Assuming the brain is in 100 percent

9 Holmes, Carl, "Mental Stimulators," introduction to *The Green Books, Vol. XXXVI: Palmer's Law of Life Palmer's Law of Life* (Davenport: The Palmer School Press, 1958), 18.

working order, the "electrical current" carried along those "power lines" is flowing at 100 percent efficiency, carrying signals along the nervous system to dictate function and to receive information. In a healthy body, the organs and muscles receive those signals, obey the brain's instructions, operate at 100 percent capacity, and report back to the brain without interference.[10]

Your nerves don't *look* very much like power lines, and they are a lot more flexible. In fact, they look a bit like stretched bubble gum. If all the nerves in your nervous system were taken out and laid end to end, they would measure *forty-five miles* long. Every one of them performs a different function in your body.

So where are these forty-five miles of nerves located? You guessed it. They exit your brain through the brain stem and travel right down your spinal cord, protected by the hard, bony armor of your vertebrae.

At various places along your spine, nerves branch off from the main bundle of the spinal cord through tiny openings in the vertebrae called spinal foramen. Stephenson explains it in his *Chiropractic Textbook* in the following way:

> *"The Spinal Cord is a bundle of nerve axons . . . a main cable to conduct mental forces from and to the brain. . . . Its branches, the spinal nerves, emit through the intervertebral foramina and ramify to all parts of the body."*[11]

Basically, what this means is that your nerves travel from your brain down your spine and carry messages to and from the rest of your body.

---

[10] Palmer, B.J., *The Green Books, Vol. XXXVI: Palmer's Law of Life* (Davenport: The Palmer School Press, 1958), 62–65.
[11] Stephenson, *Chiropractic Textbook*, 162–163.

But what happens if the messages are interfered with somewhere along the way—interrupted by those subluxations D.D. Palmer discovered back in 1895?

> *"Everything, every thing, in man lives because of intelligent energy being directed in its flow from [the] brain flowing from above-down, inside-out to its body below."*[12]
>
> —*B.J. Palmer*

If something interferes with the signals being sent by your brain, it means the current being carried by your nerves is reduced.[13] Sticking with the power line example, think of a subluxation as a tree branch falling on the lines. The signal gets reduced. When the lights go out in your house, there is usually nothing wrong with the power plant sending the energy. It's the interference that's to blame.

The power plant is still operating at 100 percent. There is usually nothing wrong with the power lines, either; they are still operating at 100 percent, too. But because of external stress being placed on the system (the pressure of a heavy tree branch against the lines) only *part* of the power being sent will arrive at its intended destination. The power gets interrupted, and the electricity on the receiving end flickers or goes out.

Now, let me pose a scenario. Let's say your medical doctor does an examination and tells you that your liver is operating at only 75 percent of its intended capacity. He might give the condition a name, known as a diagnosis.

Warning: Don't be mystified by the diagnosis. A diagnosis is, by definition, simply a made-up word used to describe symptoms. Basically, doctors use diagnoses because "cirrhosis" sounds more

---

12 Palmer, *Palmer's Law of Life*, 65.
13 Palmer, *Palmer's Law of Life*, 62–65.

professional than "your liver ain't working so good, pal." (Everything sounds more professional in Latin.)

For our purposes, we'll just call it what it is: Your liver isn't doing 25 percent of what it's supposed to do. What will your doctor do to fix this? He will probably give you some kind of medicine that instructs your liver to increase its function to make up for that missing 25 percent. Doctors do this because it produces results. The drugs administered will increase the liver's function. The problem is, the treatment doesn't really address *why* the organ isn't operating properly, and neither does the diagnosis, for that matter. Ask your doctor *why* your liver isn't working right, and the standard response will be something like, "It could be for any number of reasons, but the important thing is to get it under control. I'm going to prescribe. . . ."

The underlying assumption is that the organ is to blame, so drugs are taken to compensate for it. From now on, you just have to live with your "bad liver," (or "bad back" or "bad heart"—just fill in the blank), and you will have to take drugs for the foreseeable future to function normally.

This raises some questions. Your liver didn't always operate at 75 percent, did it? Why does your liver no longer know how to do what it is supposed to do? *What happened?* There must be a reason it stopped working normally.

Reduced Nerve Flow Equals Reduced Body Function

Organs and muscles only do what the brain tells them to do. The "power plant" of your brain sends its messages with 100 percent efficiency, regardless of the interferences between it and the recipient. But if only 75 percent of the "electrical current" actually gets through, your organs and muscles receive only 75 percent of the messages sent by your brain. In other words, 25 percent of the intended messages are lost somewhere along the way. Meanwhile, your brain carries on, not knowing that your organs and muscles are only doing 75 percent of what it is *trying* to tell them to do.[14]

This is exactly what happens when a nerve gets impinged. As R.W. Stephenson puts it, "When a nerve is 'impinged,' it means that one or more of the axons is impinged, and there is interference with transmission in the nerve."[15]

We know that impinged nerves can cause numbness and pain and can interfere with muscles' ability to contract or relax properly. Why would it be any different for your organs?

When interference occurs between your brain and your organs, chemical imbalances occur in your glands (as discussed back in Chapter One). Other organs, responding to the imbalance, alter *their* function in an attempt to compensate for the problem. One by one, parts of the body attempt to adapt, and the system is thrown into disarray, producing **SYMPTOMS**.

> **SYMPTOM: Your body's way of telling you something is wrong.**

All of this is the result of nerve interference. The medical model assumes that your organs are at fault. Doctors use medicine to alter the function of the organs and/or to diminish your symptoms.[16] Unfortunately, this model doesn't actually *fix* the problem; it only attempts to dull or compensate for symptoms. It provides temporary relief but not lasting change.

Chiropractic dismisses the idea that the organs are at fault. Instead, the chiropractic model says that reduced function is due to interference in the messages being sent from the brain to the organs (or muscles). Those interferences can be caused when misalignments

---

[14] Palmer, *Palmer's Law of Life*, 62–65.
[15] Stephenson, *Chiropractic Textbook*, 163.
[16] Palmer, *Palmer's Law of Life*, 91.

of the spinal vertebrae place pressure on your nerves. D.D. Palmer named those misalignments **VERTEBRAL SUBLUXATIONS**. In the "tree branch and power line" analogy, a subluxation is the branch, and reduced nerve flow is the interrupted electrical power.

If right now you are thinking to yourself that this all sounds incredibly simple, you are right. It's common sense! In fact, the chiropractic principle is so ridiculously simple that B.J. Palmer wrote in the introduction to his *Law of Life*, "One just criticism that can be painfully made against this book is, we repeat and repeat, and keep on repeating the same central theme until its repetition becomes boresome. We admit this fault. This New Law of Life we tell *is so simple* that once should suffice."[17]

Educating people about the vertebral subluxation and its effects is what chiropractic *was founded on*. Most people don't even know what a subluxation is, let alone that they are probably walking around subluxated right now! So forgive me for repeating myself, but it's my job to hammer this message home.

The Cause of Vertebral Subluxations

Vertebral subluxations happen when we experience physical stress, and a vertebra moves into an incorrect position and stays there. This can be such a slight injury that many people don't even realize it has happened to them. You might feel some pain at first, but the human body is made to adapt. It is so good at adapting, in fact, that the muscles and soft tissues in your spine surrounding the affected area will quickly change to match the new position, so that within a few days, most of the pain goes away.

Problem solved, right?

Not quite.

---

[17] Palmer, *Palmer's Law of Life*, 15.

When a vertebra is in the incorrect position, it means the spinal nerves exiting the intervertebral foramina are *also* now in an incorrect position. Anytime that happens, some percentage of the messages they carry becomes lost in transit.

As we have discussed, a subluxation is "the condition of a vertebra that has lost its proper juxtaposition with the one above or the one below, or both; to an extent less than a luxation; which impinges nerves and interferes with the transmission of mental impulses."[18] We're basically talking about a near-dislocation of the central nervous system's ability to communicate with the body!

The other classic example is to compare nerve flow to water in a garden hose. When a hose is flowing normally, it is not always completely filled. Minor dents in the hose—or minor subluxations— might only be noticeable at times when an extra amount of current is needed, likes times of duress when there are high levels of stress on the system, or when you're pushing yourself a little too hard.

But when the pressure on a nerve gets so bad that normal, natural flow can't get through, even in ordinary circumstances, that is when real, noticeable problems start to occur.

The danger of a subluxation is its potential "to insult the nervous system to the extent that it retards the vivification or the life-giving processes of the body."[19] The human body has the amazing power to adapt and heal itself, but a subluxated body is robbed of that full capacity. If nerves are being squeezed or pinched, the pressure "reduces [the] quantity of flow of mental impulse supply from that point outwardly going to an individual organ."[20] That's what causes "bad" organs. The organ isn't bad; it's just not getting the signals from your brain! How can you blame the organ for that? That would be

---

[18] Stephenson, *Chiropractic Textbook*, 2.
[19] Williams, Sid E., *The Meadowlands Experience* (Smyrna: Life Foundation, Inc., 1989), 23.
[20] Palmer, *Palmer's Law of Life*, 72.

like blaming the lightbulbs when the power in your house goes out! Or blaming the flowers because the garden hose stopped working.

Put simply, a subluxated body is not healing. Pressure on the nervous system leads to interference, which leads to a multitude of problems that can range from headaches to asthma to seizures to mental disorders to just about any other symptom you can think of. Have you ever visited a psychiatric hospital? That's what subluxations do to people.

And if you don't believe me yet, read on.

The Atlas: The Key to Human Health

Until you started reading this book, you were probably under the impression that 100 percent of your brain was encased in your skull, right? But as we've learned, a vital portion of it is housed in your upper cervical spine, encircled by the ATLAS and the AXIS.

The title of this book is *the* question that is *the* key to human health. The atlas is the mother lode. I tell patients and friends and audiences everywhere I go that we could literally change the *entire world* if we could just help people understand the importance of the question, "HOW'S YOUR ATLAS?"

The medulla oblongata is the part of the brain stem that serves as the connection between the brain and spinal cord. It controls your heart rate, breathing, and many other nervous system functions. It also happens to be partially encased within your atlas.

> If you have a subluxation in your atlas, there is pressure on your brain stem—literally direct pressure on your brain.

A subluxated atlas puts physical pressure on the medulla oblongata, which is just part of the reason the upper cervical region is so important. In fact, B.J. Palmer once said the atlas and the axis are the **ONLY** places where true vertebral subluxation occurs.[21] When one of those little bones is out of alignment, even by millimeters, it puts pressure on the brain stem. That is devastating to your body—and your mind.

In addition to all the potential problems caused by interfered nerve flow, we also know that pressure on the medulla insula can manifest in the form of mental illness. That is the reason my brother Ronnie and others like him started presenting symptoms of mental illness after sustaining trauma to his upper cervical spine.

The atlas is the niche that chiropractic serves. It is the source of what we do. You could be a skinny vegetarian in perfect health, but if this little bone is out of alignment a millimeter or more, you're screwed.

Given everything we've covered so far, you can understand why principled chiropractors like me get upset when we get reduced to the status of neck pain doctors or "back crackers." Chiropractic is about life! Because it doesn't matter if you're an Olympic athlete in the best shape of your life. If your atlas is subluxated, you are actively dying.

What Does a Chiropractic Adjustment Do?

"Well, okay," you might say. "So one of my vertebrae might be slightly misaligned, which might be putting a tiny bit of pressure on a few nerves. Big deal. What's the worst that can happen?"

Maybe nothing. At first. But think about it in terms of your entire lifetime. Compound those effects.

Think of all the physical stress your body has been through in your life. All the times you fell on your ass as a baby. All those spills on the playground. All the hours spent playing sports or doing physical labor

---

[21] Palmer, *Palmer's Law of Life*, 126.

or even just sitting in an incorrect posture. All the times you slept in the wrong position and woke up with a stiff neck (which is *not* normal, by the way). Many people have been subluxated since the day a doctor grabbed them by the head, twisted, wrenched, and pulled them into this world. The effects of a *major* subluxation may be obvious right away, but if it is not so major, it could take years for the manifestation to present itself.

Now, consider that human nerves are so sensitive that the *weight of a dime* is enough to disrupt nerve signals by up to 60 percent.

When you do the research, you realize that a "tiny" amount of pressure on your nervous system is not so tiny.

***

When you go to a medical doctor's office with a health issue, he or she looks for something external that is causing the internal problem—sometimes, anyway. Most of the time, your medical doctor won't even look for a cause. Nine times out of ten, they listen to your symptoms, enter them into a computer, and prescribe you whatever major medicine is currently being recommended for easing those symptoms. On another day, in another office, you might get something else. You enter the office hoping to learn what's wrong with you, and you leave with a drug and no greater understanding of why your symptoms are present in the first place. "Take two of these—and *don't* call me in the morning." Welcome to health care in America.

> "Where, how and why did THAT SOMETHING go wrong which created 'aches and pains' we think must be subdued by drugging? . . . Instead of doubling [the] inside burden by addition of drugs from [the] outside, in addition to disease inside, suppose we make it possible for THAT

> SOMETHING *inside to correct that which is*
> *wrong inside?"*[22]
>
> —*B.J. Palmer*

When something goes wrong *within* the human body, why is it we automatically believe the correct solution is to introduce some foreign substance from outside?

As Dr. Palmer put it, a logical man would realize, "If it **WAS** normal at one time, without **OUTSIDE** remedial interferences, why can't it be normal again, directing normal control **FROM INSIDE?**"[23] You could take a drug to dull your pain, to compensate for a chemical imbalance, or to do any number of other things for any number of other reasons, but all you are really doing is spinning plates—doing your best to keep up with the symptoms of problems you can't see. You're not *correcting* anything.

The goal of health shouldn't be to just dull symptoms. Symptoms are there to tell us when something is wrong. They are communicating an underlying problem. Correcting **THE CAUSE** of the problem should be the goal of health care. More often than most people realize, the cause is pressure on the nervous system.

Is there a way to correct this underlying cause? Is there a practical way to remove pressure on the nervous system?

Yes. It's called a **CHIROPRACTIC ADJUSTMENT.**

> **A chiropractic adjustment removes pressure on the nervous system and frees the nervous system to function as intended.**

The chiropractic adjustment is very easy to explain. A chiropractor, knowing the correct position of every human vertebra

---

22 Palmer, *Palmer's Law of Life*, 121.
23 Palmer, *Palmer's Law of Life*, 121.

and its ideal juxtaposition to the adjoining vertebrae, will examine your spine by touch. Through this examination, we are able to determine when vertebrae are misaligned, slightly rotated, or subluxated.

If there is no subluxation, we do not adjust you. There is no reason to.

If there is a subluxation, with your permission, we will gently and safely move the vertebra back into its correct placement. Based on your needs, this movement might be a push, or it might be a rotation. It might make a noise, or it might not. You might feel the movement, or you might not—either way, it will not be painful. Most patients agree that it feels good.

And that's it. That is all we do. Simple adjustments with our bare hands.

> *"The chiropractic principle and practice, with vertebral adjustment by hand only, permits 100 percent transmission from above-down inside-out into the assembly line."*[24]
>
> —B.J. Palmer

> *"Adjustment does not add any material or forces to the body but allows Innate to restore to normal what it would have had, had there been no interference. In this manner, health is restored."*[25]
>
> —R.W. Stephenson

[24] Palmer, *Palmer's Law of Life*, 131.
[25] Stephenson, *Chiropractic Textbook*, 2.

The chiropractic adjustment is the greatest innovation in health care since the discovery of the pulse.[26] The upper cervical spine, specifically the atlas, is the key to human health, and chiropractic adjustments are *the* way to care for it.[27] Adjustments not only have the potential to remove pressure on the brain stem and reduce nerve interference, but they are the *most practical* way to do it![28]

> *"As mental impulse flow increases and inclines, life increases and inclines, and dis-ease decreases and declines. . . . As electrical flow INCREASES AND INCLINES, light INCREASES, and darkness FADES OUT."*[29]
>
> —*B.J. Palmer*

Through a simple adjustment with the hands, we can "lift the branch off the power line," so to speak, freeing up the signals to move on through, and allowing the current to function at its natural, 100 percent capacity. This natural flow allows the body to heal itself, restoring ease to muscles and organs without drugs, surgery, or any other invasive procedures.

Life just isn't right if you're subluxated. When you are subluxated, the power of life within you gets dropped. People all around us are dying from pressure on their necks. Their brain stems are being choked off. The "current" cannot get through those power lines the way it is supposed to, and the lights are dimming, fading, and going out.

No one wants their power dropped. No one wants their baby's power dropped. We want what is best for ourselves and our loved

---

[26] Williams, *The Meadowlands Experience*, 24.
[27] Price, Galen R., "Occipito-Atlanto-Axial Region," in *Chiropractic Textbook*, Stephenson, (Davenport: The Palmer School of Chiropractic, 1948), 400.
[28] Williams, *The Meadowlands Experience*, 17.
[29] Palmer, *Palmer's Law of Life*, 64.

ones. This is why principled chiropractors are so insanely passionate about what they do. By adjusting the atlas, we can literally remove *pressure on your brain*. What other profession can claim to do that? No one. No other process short of cutting a person open can physically affect the brain. And we can do it with our bare hands, gently and painlessly, in a matter of seconds.

That was the discovery made by D.D. Palmer when he reduced the strange bump in Harvey Lillard's back, restoring a deaf man's hearing almost entirely by accident.

The effects of the vertebral subluxation are provable based on millions of other cases where function and performance in the body have been restored following a chiropractic adjustment.[30] In the next chapter, we'll talk about how and why this works, based on the processes of life, death, healing, and the innate power within the human body.

---

[30] Palmer, *Palmer's Law of Life*, 45.

Chapter 5

Innate Power

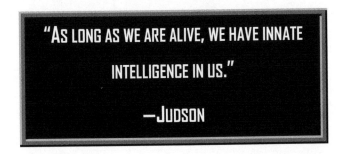

"AS LONG AS WE ARE ALIVE, WE HAVE INNATE INTELLIGENCE IN US."

—JUDSON

Chiropractic is based on the big ideas that the brain controls the body and the body can heal itself. Both of these processes occur innately.

Most processes in the human body are completely innate to us; when a baby is born, it knows how to breastfeed. It sometimes takes some practice to get it just right, but the baby knows what it's supposed to be doing—it will suckle on anything that gets near it! The newborn body knows how to take in sustenance, how to keep what it needs, and how to excrete what it doesn't. Nobody has to teach a baby how to eat... or how to poop. (Trust me. I've got five kids, remember? I should know.) Nobody has to teach a baby's body how to heal, either. Of course, there are times when certain conditions within the body and limitations of matter require outside medical intervention, but if a baby gets a scratch, that scratch is going to heal on its own!

In chiropractic, we have a name for this: **INNATE INTELLIGENCE**.

Innate Intelligence: The Process of Life

> "*INNATE REGULATES ALL. It is that abstract, intangible, unseen, perfect, immaculate, infinite and infallible regulatory factor [in] all times, all ways.*"[31]
>
> —*B.J. Palmer*

Innate literally means "born within." It's not a mystical or metaphysical thing—all it really means is that your body possesses what it needs to live.

The old chiropractors used to use the following example: If you cut your arm right now, what would happen? Blood will flow from the wound, for a start. White blood cells will quickly multiply. Before long, the blood will coagulate and clot, scabbing over to close the wound off from the environment. If the cut is very deep, puss will be produced to help stave off infection. Then the wound begins the process of healing. This process begins in the deepest part of the cut first and works its way outward until the scab falls off, revealing freshly grown skin underneath. During this process, you might cover the cut with a bandage. You might take a painkiller if it really hurts. In extreme cases, a doctor might need to sew up the cut with a few stitches or even pack the wound full of antibiotics as an extra precaution.

Now, what if you went down to the morgue and made the same cut on a dead body? What would happen? No blood would flow, that's for sure, but we could still pack the wound with antibiotics, stitch it up, and cover it with a bandage. Those things heal wounds, right? So, won't the cut heal?

---

[31] Palmer, *Palmer's Law of Life*, 24.

It's obviously impossible for a dead body to heal. It will never heal again. The life within it—its innate intelligence—has been cut off permanently. When life is gone, the body can't heal, so it dies.

> **Medicine doesn't heal you. Your body heals you.**

When I say "medicine doesn't heal you," I don't mean medicine doesn't *work*. It does work! Drugs are effective at doing what they say they do on the bottle, and if there's one thing modern medicine is good at, it is providing emergency care. Hospitals these days are extremely skilled at doing that. But when you become convinced that medicine is what heals the body, what you're essentially saying is, "This pill is what's keeping me alive, not the life within me."

In reality, medicine is only there to give your body a break and allow it the chance to heal *itself*. Somewhere along the line, we lost sight of that.

As long as we are alive, we have innate intelligence inside us. It starts in the brain and works above-down, inside-out to communicate with every cell in the body, telling every tissue, organ, and bodily process when and how to work. When innate intelligence is cut off from the body, we die (but I'll get back to that in a minute).

There is far more I could say about innate intelligence, but for now, let's address what happens when innate intelligence is *partially* cut off from the body, resulting not in death but in a state of living that is not conducive to healing—a state of *reduced life*.

> **INNATE INTELLIGENCE is the set of instructions that allows your body to function as intended.**

Ease and Dis-ease

Have you ever wondered why there are obese people who manage to live to ripe old ages, while there are also vegetarian marathon runners who drop dead of heart attacks long before their time? Why do these things happen? Luck of the draw?

Not quite.

The reason is this: You can do absolutely everything right for your entire life as far as diet and exercise are concerned, but a subluxation can still kill you.

Originally, the word "disease" meant simply a state when the body is not at ease (*ease*, plus the prefix *dis*, meaning the absence of ease). Over the course of centuries of medical science, "disease" became a term to describe specific sicknesses, infections, and the like. In our modern interpretation of disease and health care, we tend to forget there's even such a thing as "**EASE**."

In chiropractic, we say that when the body is not at ease, it is at "**DIS-EASE**." B.J. Palmer defined dis-ease as "destroyed functional activity."[32] In his *Law of Life*, he said, "Dis-ease is an intermediate declining stage somewhere between life and death."[33]

Stephenson puts it the following way:

> *"DISEASE is a term used by physicians for sickness. To them it is an entity that one can have and is worthy of a name, hence diagnosis. DIS-EASE is a term used in chiropractic, meaning not having ease. . . . In chiropractic, EASE is the entity, and dis-ease is the lack of it. Dis-ease, in chiropractic, is indicative of the*

[32] Palmer, *Palmer's Law of Life*, 79.
[33] Palmer, *Palmer's Law of Life*, 64.

> *body being minus something that should be*
> *restored, in order to make it normal."*[34]
>
> —R.W. Stephenson

> *"The cause of dis-ease is interference with*
> *transmission of mental impulses. The*
> *subluxation is the physical representation of the*
> *cause. Interference with transmission causes dis-*
> *ease by preventing Innate from producing*
> *adaptation in the tissue cell; hence it becomes*
> *unsound and not at ease."*[35]
>
> —R.W. Stephenson

Basically, by the contemporary definition, a disease is something you can catch or acquire somehow; it is something *getting in* that shouldn't be there. Dis-ease, on the other hand, according to the definition of the principled chiropractor, is a manifestation of an underlying problem. It is something that *should be* there that is not being expressed correctly because of an interference.

Now, back to death. . . .

Paralysis of Action: The Process of Death

What is death, really? How do we define it? Let's say you didn't have a bunch of fancy medical equipment and sensors and beeping

---

34 Stephenson, *Chiropractic Textbook*, 80.
35 Stephenson, *Chiropractic Textbook*, 82.

heart monitors to tell that a person was alive. How would you be able to tell when they were dead?

The answer is not all that mysterious. All of the things that we identify as signifying death (lack of a heartbeat, no pulse, the stoppage of breathing, and the absence of brain function) all boil down to one simple thing: **MOVEMENT!**[36]

As B.J. Palmer once put it, "There is only **ONE** dis-ease, regardless of where or what organ or organs involved: **PARALYSIS OF ACTION.**"[37] Movement means life. If any of the above-mentioned indicators of life are still present (still moving), it means there is still life left in the body. When none of those factors are present (paralysis of action), it means the body is no longer a suitable habitat for life, so life has left the body. The body is dead.

When someone is subluxated, their "normal function" decreases until it becomes "abnormal function." That leads to "minus function," and then "paralysis." Paralysis of any part of the body leads to dis-ease, the breakdown of health, and eventually, total paralysis—death.[38] The process looks like this:

1. Normal function
2. Vertebral subluxation
3. Nerve interference
4. Abnormal function
5. Minus function
6. Paralysis
7. Dis-ease
8. Death

The "paralysis of action" B.J. Palmer talked about begins when a vertebral subluxation interrupts normal function. A person who is 100 percent healthy is functioning normally, while a dead body is at

---

[36] Palmer, *Palmer's Law of Life*, 63.
[37] Palmer, *Palmer's Law of Life*, 122.
[38] Stephenson, *Chiropractic Textbook*, 206.

zero percent. Sick people—and let's face it, that probably accounts for most of us—are somewhere between 100 percent and zero.[39]

Earlier, I posed a scenario where only 75 percent of electrical current made it through the interference caused by a branch on the power lines. But what happens if things get *really* bad? What if it's such a heavy branch—or so many individual branches, in multiple locations—that only 50 percent of nerve transmission gets through to your body? Or 25 percent?

Or zero?

It's simple. When the current being sent from your brain is too greatly disrupted and an organ can't function at all anymore (because it doesn't know how), the lights go off permanently. There's a technical term for this: kicking the bucket.

Most people spend their entire lives in a steady nosedive toward zero percent nerve transmission. At the point when our bodies are no longer capable of functioning as intended, and we are no longer a suitable habitat for life, life "takes a prolonged vacation—called death."[40] The body cannot adjust to its environment or its internal conditions, and life ceases to flow within it. Ashes to ashes, dust to dust.

> *"Life is one hundred percent function; perfect coordination; absolute adaptation. Death is zero percent function; absence of coordination; total lack of adaptation, which brings the matter of the body under the sway of universal forces, the same as any other 'dust.'"*[41]
>
> —R.W. Stephenson

---

39 Palmer, *Palmer's Law of Life*, 63.
40 Palmer, *Palmer's Law of Life*, 42.
41 Stephenson, *Chiropractic Textbook*, 206.

You now know the exact progression of sickness: the breakdown of the body's natural state of ease. It begins with a vertebral subluxation, leading to nerve interference, followed by abnormal function, minus function, paralysis, dis-ease, and death.

The question you should now be asking is, can we stop this process? I'll do you one better. We can not only stop this process—we can *reverse* it.

Chapter 6

Retracing: The Journey Continues

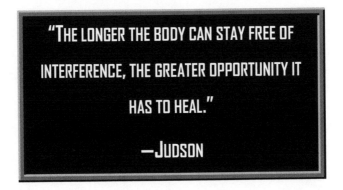

> "THE LONGER THE BODY CAN STAY FREE OF INTERFERENCE, THE GREATER OPPORTUNITY IT HAS TO HEAL."
>
> —JUDSON

Ronnie Judson's nosedive toward zero percent nerve transmission began the day a 285-pound lineman snapped his neck. No one disagreed with the fact that all my brother's mental health problems all coincided with his neck injury, but no doctor had ever suggested to us that there was any connection.

Years had gone by since the accident. I was working my way through chiropractic school, and given everything I had learned so far, I realized that the problems Ronnie had developed were textbook symptoms of a subluxation in the upper cervical region. Everything about my brother's story pointed to a massive subluxation that had put pressure on his brain stem. Over time, that pressure impaired his mental function, and things kept getting progressively worse.

The things I learned from Dr. Kale at DE, plus the knowledge I gained at Life University, led me to conclude that Ronnie *could* get help. He might never return to the person he used to be, but the ongoing mental deterioration could at least stop. Some of his problems might even be reversed!

Chiropractic Fails Ronnie Judson . . . Again

I wasn't a chiropractor yet, so I couldn't provide the care Ronnie needed. But I tracked down a man who was a master at providing adjustments in the upper cervical region. (For the sake of this book and for reasons you'll soon understand, this chiropractor will remain nameless.)

This chiropractor agreed to see my brother, so I drove home to New York, snuck Ronnie out of the halfway house he was living in at the time, and drove him all the way down to the Carolinas to get Ronnie adjusted by this chiropractor. Then we drove to Georgia so he could stay with me while I was going to school.

For two weeks, I drove Ronnie from Georgia to the Carolinas every day. It was expensive, but I could already see him changing—after just two weeks! He was actually getting better, and for the first time in a long time, we had hope.

Then we ran out of money.

Ronnie was responding great to the adjustments, but this chiropractor was very expensive. Two weeks under his care was all my family could afford.

I approached the guy and explained the situation. I asked if there was any way we could work something out so that Ronnie could stay under his care. I asked if we could arrange a payment plan. Or maybe I could do some extra work in his office on the weekends. I even offered to come and work for him full-time after I graduated chiropractic school to work off the cost.

His answer was no. No price reduction. No payment plan. No working off the cost. No deal. Basically, if my family didn't have the money, he said we couldn't afford him.

That was it. We were cut off.

I had no other options. I had to take Ronnie back to the halfway house in New York. Soon, he started to deteriorate all over again. They had to put him back in an institution, and they doped him up as usual.

Money. Fucking *money* prevented my brother from getting his life back. It's not like I expected this nameless chiropractor to work for free. I would have been willing to work out any deal he wanted. But he wouldn't budge. A man who claimed to have devoted himself to getting people well decided to leverage the chiropractic principle for money.

Obviously, I was pissed. But I wasn't just angry at that chiropractor. I found myself wishing, "God, why couldn't there have been someone around who knew about chiropractic the day Ronnie got hurt?"

There were probably a hundred other people on the field for practice the day Ronnie was hit. Not one of them knew about chiropractic care? The more I thought about it, the more impossible I realized that was. I'm sure the coaches and trainers on the sidelines had seen neck injuries before. But not one of them told my brother to go see a chiropractor.

What about all our friends and neighbors and classmates? Ronnie was practically a legend in my hometown! *Everyone* had heard the story of what happened to him. Thousands of people. People he played with, people he went to school with, people who looked up to him or just followed him in sports—you mean to tell me none of them had ever heard about chiropractic?

What about all the professors who saw the changes in his grades and his attitude after his injury? What about all the specialists my parents took him to see? What about the doctors at the hospitals and institutions? You mean to tell me not one of them knew he might benefit from chiropractic care?

I am willing to bet at least one chiropractor heard Ronnie's story at one point or another. But did they take the time to reach out to my family? No. If they had—if anyone had offered any possibility of hope—we would have jumped at it. We were desperate! But they didn't reach out. They just didn't take the time.

In hindsight, knowing what I know now, my brother's story is even more tragic. I know deep in my heart that if my brother had received proper care after his injury, the whole process could have been reversed. It pisses me off to know that someone out there must have known the truth and could have stood up and said something, but they didn't.

Ronnie could have gotten his life back.

***

My hard work at Life University paid off. Despite being a crappy student for most of my academic career, I passed my boards, graduated, and earned a Doctorate of Chiropractic. God is good.

I now knew what I had been put on this earth to do, and I was ready to go out and do it. I was training, reading, studying, interviewing, talking to doctors, going to their offices, traveling around the world on mission trips, going to orphanages and psychiatric hospitals and prisons. . . . I didn't watch TV for seven years. I was too busy.

I committed myself to learning the procedure Ronnie had been denied, because I was going to learn it, become the best at it, and make it affordable. I would bring this thing to the masses and help people who couldn't get help anywhere else. People like Ronnie and families like mine.

I trained with Dr. Kale for six years. I went to Russia with him. Over time, I learned the specialized upper cervical procedure he used.

At this point in the story, people usually ask me, did you bring Ronnie? What happened to Ronnie? To understand the answer to that question, I need to explain two key concepts: momentum and retracing.

Momentum and Retracing

"Momentum is the possession of motion; requiring effort and time to stop it. Chiropractically, momentum is the progress of dis-ease or health, requiring time and effort to stop it." [42]

—R.W. Stephenson

A lot of patients feel better *immediately* after receiving a single chiropractic adjustment, and major symptoms that have been bothering them may start to reduce after a few adjustments. That's the power of relieving pressure on the nervous system. But it's not an instantaneous fix. Underlying problems take longer to address. The body needs time to heal itself, and we need to be persistent about making sure the atlas is clear and that pressure on the nervous system is not present.

The longer the body can stay free of interference, the greater opportunity it has to heal—to bounce back from dis-ease, recover, regain that natural state of ease, and restore health. We call this process "retracing." [43]

---

42 Stephenson, *Chiropractic Textbook*, 96.
43 Stephenson, *Chiropractic Textbook*, 98.

> *"Every case [of dis-ease] retraces, for if there is a departure from health, there must be a return to it, if there is restoration. When a case retraces, it passes back through the successive steps, in reverse order, that it passed through in getting worse."*[44]
>
> —R.W. Stephenson

Retracing is the reason it takes time for sick people to get well. It's the reason your body doesn't automatically, magically return to 100 percent ease after a single chiropractic adjustment. And it's the reason most chiropractors suggest that their patients return for follow-up appointments.

Those follow-up appointments have become a source of contention in our profession. A lot of cynical people suspect chiropractors of telling people to come back all the time just because it's good for business. News flash: We are doctors. That is not how doctors operate. Return appointments are not a money-making scheme. Consistent care is the way we keep your nervous system clear so that your body can heal. To suggest that we do it just to make a little extra cash is insulting to everything we stand for.

I can tell you from experience—and millions of people under chiropractic care will back me up on this—that the people who do come back get awesome results. When their nervous systems stay clear, they heal. Meanwhile, the people who decide not to come back next week because they think the chiropractor's just trying to squeeze a few extra bucks out of them . . . a lot of times, they end up coming back anyway. But instead of one week later, it's one month later. Or six months later. Or a year. They come back when the pain is so bad they can barely stand or when they wake up and their neck is so stiff they

---

44 Stephenson, *Chiropractic Textbook*, 98.

can't turn their head. Remember when I said the weight of a dime can reduce nerve transmission by 60 percent? If agonizing pain and dysfunction are manifesting themselves outwardly, can you imagine what is going on in the nervous system, underneath it all?

People who decide that regular care isn't important often come back worse than ever. By neglecting their nervous system health, their bodies have deteriorated back to a state of chronic dis-ease. Every chiropractor has patients like this, and when they come back, we do what we always do: We examine them, give them the adjustment they need for a little relief, and tell them to come back for a follow-up appointment. And, big surprise, they often don't listen . . . and the cycle starts all over again.

If those people just took our recommendations instead of being so suspicious of us, they wouldn't be in such bad shape. People wouldn't need to come to the chiropractor for emergency situations for relief from unbearable pain if they would just come in regularly.

It pisses me off that people get suspicious of chiropractors, thinking that we're just trying to make a buck. We are trying to help. We are trying to heal you!

You want to talk about money? How about the expensive prescription drugs your doctor prescribes to treat your diagnosis? For drug companies, a prescription is guaranteed income for life—*your* life, anyway. For you, it's a guaranteed expense until the day you die. And you're upset because the chiropractor wants you to come back in two weeks? Which option do you think will cost you more in the long run?

In the ideal situation, there is no need for retracing. If you can make sure your atlas is clear *before* problems arise, your body does not have to go through the stress of trying to heal itself from all the compounded effects of subluxations. In Ronnie's case, things had been so bad for so long that it would be a massive uphill battle.

Chapter 7

The Symptom Mentality and the Folly of Drugs

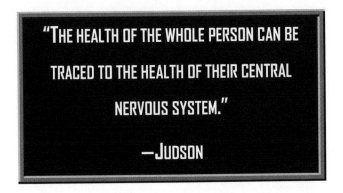

"THE HEALTH OF THE WHOLE PERSON CAN BE TRACED TO THE HEALTH OF THEIR CENTRAL NERVOUS SYSTEM."

—JUDSON

"A physical or mental feature that is regarded as indicating a condition or disease." What you have just read is the definition of the word **SYMPTOM**.

A symptom is basically a bodily state indicative of an underlying cause. When you have symptoms like aches and pains, it means your body is trying to tell you that *something is wrong*. If your response is to immediately reach for relief in the form of a bottle of pills, you are not addressing what is wrong. All you're doing is numbing symptoms, which means you will never know why those symptoms were there in the first place; you're ignoring the underlying problem.

Here's a famous example offered up by B.J. Palmer in his book *Palmer's Law of Life*, similar to the garden hose analogy we used earlier. If a farmer were watering his cows and attempted to use the water hose only to find that the hose was not functioning properly, what would he do? Would he just accept that the water hose, which had been functioning normally a day before, is now broken (a "bad" hose)? Or would he retrace the path of the hose to find the kink in it and fix it?

Any intelligent farmer would find the place where the hose's flow had been impinged, remove the kink, and go back to work with a fully functioning water hose. A chiropractor is like that farmer. He sees impaired performance and wants to fix it. He wants to find the source of the problem and remove it—remove the interference. Many medical doctors, on the other hand, might diagnose the hose with "trickleitis," "sputteritis," or "dribbleitis."[45] Like most diagnoses, these are unhelpful, made-up words introduced simply to describe the presence of symptoms.

> *"You go into a general practitioner; he gives you a cursory physical examination. He says, 'Go take this pill.' You come back in three weeks, and he says, 'That's not effective, go take this one.' 'Go take that one.' 'Go take this one.' Is that science?"[46]*
>
> *—Dr. Sid Williams*

> *"What does [the] average person do when he has 'aches and pains'? He takes [drugs] or some other of many forms of external medications or treatments to suppress, paralyze, deaden, dull ALL sense of flow feeling between lower efferent disease and upper brain interpretations. All [drugs] or any other external treatment does is TO COMPLETELY SHUT OFF, PARALYZE OR*

45 Palmer, *Palmer's Law of Life*, 108.
46 Williams, *The Meadowlands Experience*, 14.

> BLOCK *all sense messages traveling through nerves from organ below to brain above."*[47]
>
> —*B.J. Palmer*

A World Without Drugs

When you take a drug to deal to feel better, it does not mean you *are* better. It does not fix the problem at all. The problem that caused the pain is still going strong. In fact, the pain itself is actually still going strong, too—you just can't feel it anymore! Thanks to an unnatural chemical concoction that was never meant to be in your body, you are comfortably numb.

> *"Any substance or chemical not prepared by Innate and introduced into the body is a poison."*[48]
>
> —*R.W. Stephenson*

> *"Poison is any substance introduced into or manufactured within the living body which Innate cannot use in metabolism."*[49]
>
> —*R.W. Stephenson*

Let's say you develop a symptom. Something is not right in your body, so you visit your family doctor who refers you to a specialist.

---

47 Palmer, *Palmer's Law of Life*, 118.
48 Stephenson, *Chiropractic Textbook*, 114.
49 Stephenson, *Chiropractic Textbook*, 120.

The problem is, specialty doctors sometimes develop tunnel vision. They are trained to see patients' symptoms through the lens of their specific field. There is a good chance this specialist will recommend a prescription drug to alleviate some of your symptoms.

People who are experiencing multiple sets of symptoms often end up in the offices of multiple specialists. They follow the advice of each of these specialists and are soon taking multiple prescription drugs.

The problem is, it never occurs to anyone involved that these different sets of symptoms might be related. All of these symptoms could all be the result of *the same* underlying process, which is being completely ignored.

As a society, our thinking about health care has become overly focused on symptoms and the consultations of specialists whose tunnel vision has the potential to cloud a lot of the purpose behind why they became doctors in the first place. We have lost sight of helping the whole person. The health of the whole person can be traced to the health of their central nervous system.

> *"There IS NO LAW OF DRUGS. They come today and go tomorrow. The fad of the hour has its drug of the hour."[30]*
>
> —*B.J. Palmer*

In my version of an ideal world, there would be no drugs. I'm tempted to say something really drastic, like, "Let's throw all the drugs in the ocean." It would be a great day for humanity but a very bad day for fish.

One of the reasons I get so fired up over these sorts of things is because the use of antipsychotics on privately insured children ages two to five in the United States doubled from 1999 to 2007. According to a study in the January 2010 *Journal of the American Academy of*

---

[30] Palmer, *Palmer's Law of Life*, 109.

Child & Adolescent Psychiatry, more than 1 million children in that same age group, with private health insurance, were diagnosed with bipolar disorder.[51]

In the past ten years, that number has skyrocketed. Medicaid records in some U.S. states show that infants younger than one year old are on drugs for mental disorders. These are some of the most powerful, mind-altering drugs on the planet, and we are giving them to *babies*. The most troubling part is that the diagnosis of psychiatric disorders differs from doctor to doctor. One psychiatrist might diagnose a disorder while another might not.

Two-year-olds are being given drugs for the treatment of bipolar disorder, a condition marked by elevated moods, times of happiness and increased energy offset by times of depression and a negative outlook on life. Have you ever *met* a two-year-old? How many two-year-olds do you know with a negative outlook on life?

I know this all sounds crazy, but it is happening all the time. We are giving our own children powerful psychotropic drugs, and for what? To control the "terrible twos"?

Health Care vs. Sick-Care

I have seen firsthand that kids who have never taken drugs and have received chiropractic adjustments since day one have a next-level expression of life. Instead of going to the medical doctor when they are sick to take external drugs that numb the symptoms of internal problems, they go to a chiropractor when they are well, and they are cared for so they can *stay* well.

---

[51] Olfson, Mark, Stephen Crystal, Cecilia Huang, and Tobias Gerhard, "Trends in Antipsychotic Drug Use by Very Young, Privately Insured Children," *Journal of the American Academy of Child & Adolescent Psychiatry*, January 2010, Volume 49, Issue 1, 13–23.

I spoke earlier about the mistaken concept of "bad" organs. When an organ is not working properly, medical doctors rarely try to determine what is going on. They prescribe whichever medication claims to normalize the symptoms in question. Or better yet—just remove the organ! "The thing's not working right? No problem. We'll just chop that sucker right out of you."

These doctors are quick to offer a "fix," but they rarely attempt to attribute an organ's dysfunction to any *cause* or *process*. They treat organs as if each has a mind of its own, disconnected from the rest of the body, and when one gets out of line, they either force it to work properly or they cut it from the team—sometimes literally.

> *"Patient and doctor have lost sight of the totality of the sick person."*[52]
>
> —B.J. Palmer

The above quote by B.J. Palmer was written in 1958, and things have gotten far worse since then.

It is time to change this mindset. People need to stop mindlessly inundating their own bodies with poisons and start taking their health back!

> *"Medical practices, dealing externally with internal diseases, regard certain organs as SEPARATE, to be studied and treated as disorganized units . . . independent of all others, with no association in relation to other organs, as though it hung in selfish space and acted flagrantly from any other, or had nothing to do with relationship with any other. Therapists of*

---

[52] Palmer, *Palmer's Law of Life*, 100.

> *all kinds think of the brain, spinal cord, spinal*
> *nerves, nervous system, as though they were*
> *unbelievably independent units . . . each*
> *refusing in some distant way to be unrelated to*
> *the balance of the anatomical and physiological*
> *body."*[33]
>
> —*B.J. Palmer*

Ronnie Judson Today

> *"We can exist 40 days without foods. We can*
> *navigate 40 hours without fluids. But, we can't*
> *live 40 minutes without mental impulse supply*
> *flowing freely from above-down, inside out,*
> *brain to body."*[34]
>
> —*B.J. Palmer*

Ultimately, it was too late for Ronnie Judson. *Everybody* can benefit from chiropractic care at *any* point in their lives, no matter what state of health they are in; there is always hope for a better life. But the effects of a subluxation are compounded over time, meaning that the longer it goes unadjusted, the worse it gets and the longer and more difficult it becomes to retrace.

In Ronnie's case, we were dealing with a devastating subluxation in the upper cervical region—direct pressure on the brain stem that had been there for years upon years. When the nervous system is that

53 Palmer, *Palmer's Law of Life*, 96.
54 Palmer, *Palmer's Law of Life*, 61.

overtaxed for that long, even after the subluxation is corrected there simply may not be enough time left for the body to heal itself.

Things were made so much worse by the fact that Ronnie had been pumped full of drugs in the years since the injury. The body can heal itself of anything when it is clear, but he had been on so many medications for so long that his body was dependent on them. He could no longer even function without the drugs. Any hope of restoring my brother to normal health and saving his life was long gone.

I used to have these conversations with God where I would say, "Couldn't you just make it better, God? I'll give up everything I have if you can just make Ronnie normal." After a while, my prayers changed. The pain and the heartache took their toll. I started praying that Ronnie could just die peacefully at night in his sleep, so he didn't have to suffer anymore.

To this day, Ronnie is living in a halfway house in New York. He barely resembles the man he once was. He is kept constantly doped up just so his body can function. When I visit him, he smiles at me. His teeth have all rotted out because of the side effects of some of the drugs, but he smiles nonetheless. Ronnie Judson is still in there, but he's not the same. He will never be the same person again. Trapped somewhere inside that prison cell is the man who lifted me up on the baseball field all those years ago—the man who pitched no-hitters and was an inspiration to the kids in our hometown and had the strength, intelligence, and power to have changed the world if he had gotten the chance.

When I look at Ronnie's story, it breaks my heart. It kills me. He was always a better man than me. He was always stronger. He deserved a great life. Instead, everything was stolen from him.

Chiropractic failed my family. I was led on the path to become a chiropractor as a result, which I am grateful for; I just wish my brother and best friend hadn't had to lose his life for it to happen. I almost lost *my* life, too, by watching the closest person to me suffer. With a family history of alcoholism and all the things I have seen in my life, I could have ended up in a very dark place. God did not let that happen. Instead, Ronnie's story fueled my fire. It motivated me to not let this happen to somebody else. No one told my family about chiropractic when Ronnie needed it, but maybe I could be that guy for someone else.

That leads us to the big question: Are *you* subluxated?

Are You Subluxated?

Do you have constant health problems? Do you feel like you get sick more often than other people? Do you numb yourself with drugs and intoxicate your mind so you can get through everyday life? Can you hardly remember what it was like to just feel normal? Does your life seem like it "just ain't right"?

That's not living!

If I just described *you*, IT IS TIME TO SEE A CHIROPRACTOR.

You need to realize that it is *not normal* to be in pain. It is *not normal* to feel like something isn't right!

Come see a principled chiropractor. We don't heal you of anything; we simply remove the source of interference so your body can do what it naturally does: heal itself. It's not about stiff necks or lower back pain. It's about making sure your nervous system is clear. All we have to do is take that pressure off the brain stem and make sure it stays that way. The longer it stays that way, the more opportunity your body has to heal, and the greater your life will be as a result.

> *"WHAT is the principle of Chiropractic? To correct cause.*
>
> *WHERE is cause? A vertebral subluxation.*

> *WHY is vertebral subluxation THE cause? It interferes with normal quantity flow of nerve force between brain and body, from above-down, inside out.*
>
> *WHERE is vertebral subluxation located? In the occipito-atlantal-axial area, occasionally at lower areas.*
>
> *HOW do Chiropractors correct this vertebral subluxation? By adjustment, by hand only.*
>
> *HOW does this get sick well? By permitting normal restoration of normal quantity flow of mental impulse supply between brain and body. By permitting the inherent, internal Innate intellectuality and forces within body of patient [to] cure and heal from above-down, inside-out.*"[55]
>
> —B.J. Palmer

Ronnie Judson would be an amazing human being today if one knowledgeable, principled chiropractor had just laid their hands on him before it was too late. If one person could have adjusted my brother's spine and cleared it out, it could have changed the course of his life. Instead, he lost his life, and my kids missed out on having an amazing uncle all because no one shared the chiropractic story with us.

My main message to you is: **GET YOUR ATLAS CHECKED AND GET YOUR NERVOUS SYSTEM CLEAR!**

Listen to your chiropractor. He or she has your best interests at heart. If you have reason to believe they do not, consult the final

---

[55] Palmer, *Palmer's Law of Life*, 92.

chapter of this book, which discusses how to find a principled chiropractor.

Get yourself to a *principled* chiropractor. Get yourself checked and clear, and your life is going to be awesome.

***

I started my career in chiropractic with a fire in my heart that most people cannot understand. Giving my first adjustment was absolutely euphoric. I adjusted someone's atlas, and it felt like a lightning bolt passed through my body. It was one of the most powerful things I had ever experienced. After all the schooling I had gone through, all the classes and exams, to have all that training and work come together in a single moment in time.... Wow. It was one of the coolest experiences of my life, and it only served to further affirm that this was my calling.

My wife Tammy and I took the hard road. Some people have everything handed to them, but not us. (My daddy didn't give me a dime. I got a pat on the back and a wish for good luck.) We moved up north to Tammy's home state of Connecticut, and that was where I planned to open my first chiropractic office. I discovered that the state of Connecticut had some different laws for practicing chiropractic. In forty-six of the fifty United States, I could have just walked right in and started practicing, but not Connecticut. I had to wait for about a year to get my license because of the way the laws were set up. In that time, we had our first baby, Kylie. We had nothing but each other and our drive to change people's lives.

Our first practice was a 400-square-foot office. Looking back at it now, it's kind of hilarious. We grew fast—and since I didn't know what I was doing on the business end of things, it was almost painfully fast. Before we knew it, we were too big for 400 square feet. We upgraded to something a little roomier: an office space that was between 1,000 and 1,200 feet.

I was content there, but God had other plans.

I would have sworn that that second office would be enough space well into the foreseeable future, but the people just kept coming. The business kept growing.

Today, my office is more like a facility, where we see between 100 and 200 people every day. The whole process happened innately. I never even advertised until recently, but I started because I realized I had no choice. I *have* to spread the word and get more people under care, because I don't want what happened to Ronnie to happen to anybody ever again. If I have anything to say about it, it won't.

Chapter 8

Uncompromising: The Chiropractic Principle

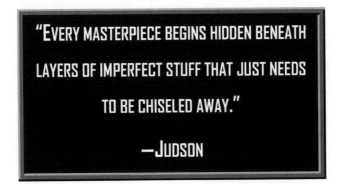

"EVERY MASTERPIECE BEGINS HIDDEN BENEATH
LAYERS OF IMPERFECT STUFF THAT JUST NEEDS
TO BE CHISELED AWAY."

—JUDSON

Chiropractic has been the target of a lot of mudslinging over the years. The established medical community has historically had problems with what we do. Decades ago, there was actually a lawsuit by chiropractors against the American Medication Association for defamation because the AMA was calling chiropractors "unscientific cultists."[56] The chiropractors *won* the case. In fact, we now know that the AMA even had a special committee dedicated to coming up with ways to undermine chiropractic.

In other words, we chiropractors know what it's like to be kicked when we're down. We know what it's like to be up against an industry that we could never hope to overcome monetarily or in terms of numbers, even though surveys say that our patients are healthy, happy, and satisfied with our services. But we can continue to win people over through the results they experience, one person at a time.

---

[56] "U.S. Judge Finds Medical Group Conspired Against Chiropractors," *The New York Times*, August 29, 1987.

> "We have so many chiropractors today that say, 'Oh, that's not scientific. We need to prove the subluxation.' I've got a simple colloquial answer to that; the French proved the subluxation in 1835 when they invented the guillotine."[57]
>
> —Dr. Sid Williams

One of my patients, shortly after her new patient orientation, brought me an article about a UPenn football player who had just hung himself. For obvious reasons, any story about a UPenn football player is going to strike a chord with me, but what was really remarkable was that the story mentioned that research being done in the mental health field is finding that pressure on the brain—like the kind that can occur in football injuries—can cause chemical imbalances in the body, which can cause depression and anxiety.

Pressure on the brain stem? Chemical imbalances? Any of that sound familiar? If not, go back to Chapter One of this book!

What they are describing is a SUBLUXATION!

These researchers are "discovering" things that chiropractors have known about for over a hundred years! And who fixes subluxations? We do. Not MDs, not physical therapists. Physical therapists are trying to learn now, but they will never perfect it like we already have. Chiropractors are masters of their craft. We are tenth-degree black belts at this stuff.

A recent study was conducted in which the researchers sought to better understand why SLEEP exists. We all understand the need for rest, but what practical need does sleep actually fulfill in the body?

---

57 Williams, *The Meadowlands Experience*, 14.

When you think about it, sleep is awfully risky. Every night, we have to leave ourselves open and totally defenseless against all kinds of potential dangers. Yet it is a requirement for all mammals and most other animals, too. Why?

The study found that rats that were forcibly deprived of sleep died within a couple of weeks. Interestingly enough, studies on sleeping rats showed an increase in the amount of cerebrospinal fluid circulating between the spine and the brain while they were asleep.

The inferred result of the study was that sleep allows the body to rest, but it also fulfills another need: The brain needs to be "cleaned" regularly as a means of maintenance, and the interchange of fluid between the spinal cord and the brain is instrumental in this. That, they believe, is why sleep is necessary to life and why animals will die if deprived of sleep for too long. This "new discovery" sounds an awful lot like what B.J. Palmer said back in 1958:

"With 100 per cent natural sleep, Innate concentrates 100 percent of focalized recuperative, reconstructive, rebuilding forces to internal physical necessities. It alone knows where, when, and how much. . . . Many people go to bed with a headache and wake up without it. That's partially what occurs."[58]

---

[58] Palmer, *Palmer's Law of Life*, 22.

> "Three to four hours of complete, natural relaxation, even to sleeping, are important following a Chiropractic adjustment. This permits Innate to focalize muscular contractions TO SET AND RESET minute micrometer relations of a subluxation beyond the ken of education, even a Chiropractor."[59]
> This sort of thing happens more often than you might think. "New" medical science proves something chiropractors have been teaching and sharing for more than a century of practice.
> When will people learn?

So many wise-asses out there try to belittle what chiropractors do. Sometimes I argue with them, but other times, I ignore them because I know it's just a waste of a conversation.

I have the certainty, day in and day out, that I am taking pressure off the nervous system. I am sold on this principle. I don't need to second-guess anything, and I don't need anybody in my life who is going to second-guess it either.

The principle of chiropractic has changed the lives of countless millions of people, and it will continue to do so. Chiropractors who are plugged into that principle of life are driven. They are passionate, and they make things happen, period. The principle is present in our offices, outside our offices, in our hearts and souls, and in every single man, woman, or child who walks our path.

> *"Chiropractic analysis is the process of finding which subluxation or subluxations to adjust,*

---

59 Palmer, *Palmer's Law of Life*, 22.

> *according to major methods . . . with the view of finding the cause.*"[60]
>
> —*R.W. Stephenson*

A Failure Story

I had a patient a couple of years ago whose story really sticks with me.

This woman (we'll call her Annie) had a tough life. Annie had two kids. Her son was in a wheelchair and couldn't even go to the bathroom on his own, and her daughter took a lot of drugs to treat the symptoms of too many health problems to count. All three became patients under my care.

Pretty soon, with regular checks and adjustments when appropriate, Annie's son started to be able to go to the bathroom on his own. Her daughter's symptoms became less severe, and we managed to get her off all those drugs. Unfortunately, all three of them stopped coming in because of some stress at home brought on by Annie's husband.

I had met Annie's husband a few times while his family was under my care. He was this big guy who worked out five or six days a week. He was in the kind of physical shape every guy wishes he could be. Annie's husband clearly made his health a priority, but each time I suggested he join his family under chiropractic care and get himself checked, he brushed off my advice. He said he didn't need it; he was a "healthy person."

By most standards, he was right. He wasn't sick. He took care of himself. He had no visible health problems or outward symptoms. He was a strong, great-looking guy who was physically fit and proud of it.

---

60 Stephenson, *Chiropractic Textbook*, 224.

"But if you're subluxated," I said, "you're not living your life to its fullest potential. You can see your family starting to thrive here. We've got to get you under care, too."

I talked to him several times about getting under chiropractic care, always with the same result. He shrugged it off and claimed he didn't need it. His reasoning was basically, "If it ain't broke, don't fix it," and I never managed to get it through his head that he should just lie down on the table and get checked.

Oh well. I tried, right? Can't win them all.

But guess what? I failed him.

One day, I got a call from Annie. She told me that she needed all her medical records for her attorney because her healthy husband had dropped dead five weeks ago from a massive heart attack. She said the doctors were bewildered. They had no answers as to why this had happened.

As an aside, there is a good chance that you will someday (if you haven't already) have to deal with a certain kind of medical doctor—the MD who does *not* like to have his or her authority questioned. You know the kind of person I'm talking about. They are arrogant. Holier than thou. Above you. Their time is precious, and they are annoyed by your questions, sometimes nearly to the point of hostility. How dare you ask a question of *them*?

And then, when something like this occurs—a fit, young man dropping dead long before his time—the same doctor will shrug his or her shoulders and say, "It's just one of those things that happens sometimes." Total lack of accountability.

I'll tell you why this happened. The guy was subluxated! By all appearances, this big, strong man was doing everything right. The one thing he wasn't doing was getting his power turned on. It doesn't matter how in-shape you are, how far you can run, how many pounds you can lift—if you are subluxated, your body's ability to produce life is impaired. He was subluxated, and in the end, it killed him.

I tried to show him the truth, and I tried to get him under care. I did everything I could, right?

Wrong!

If you ask me, I failed. I didn't push him enough. I should have tried harder, not just for his sake but for the sake of his family, too. That is on me. How's that for accountability?

Incongruent: The Rise of Unprincipled Chiropractic

"We would be derelict of our obligation to protect the sick, if we did not WARN THEM what to look for in a chiropractor's office and what to avoid."[61]

—B.J. Palmer

"Do ALL 'chiropractors' do what they should? No! Why? Because, out there in those big, wide-open spaces are multitudes of sick people. They have been educated for centuries to 'do something' to disease itself, from outside-in, below-upward. Give, inject, take, treat something internal physical with something external physical. Some 'chiropractors' (?) appease, listen to, and do what the sick have

---

[61] Palmer, *Palmer's Law of Life*, 145.

> *been taught to want, always beg for, implore*
> *and tease them to do.*[62]
>
> —B.J. Palmer

Everything I've shared with you so far has been straight from the source. The principles in this book come from D.D. Palmer (the founder of chiropractic), his son B.J. Palmer (the developer of chiropractic), and other titans of our profession who followed in their footsteps and carried on their legacies.

But sadly, there is a great divide among chiropractors. The ugly truth is that not every chiropractor embodies, practices, or even believes in the principles our philosophy is supposed to stand for. To understand why this is, you have to go back a few years, to a time when the chiropractic profession fell under poor leadership. To put it mildly, the leaders of chiropractic were a bunch of sissies. And in their rush to be "accepted," the principle was lost.

> The PRINCIPLED CHIROPRACTOR has a driving, seated passion for what he or she does. They believe in the same powerful principles that have been handed down since the beginning.

In previous chapters, I've shared the principles of chiropractic in detail. By now, you know that the subluxation and the adjustment are at the core of what we do, but I can't tell you how many times I get patients from other chiropractors' offices who have *never been adjusted* before. Instead, they have been poked and prodded, massaged and stretched. I'll admit, they have some pretty flexible hamstrings, but stretches don't correct subluxations!

---

[62] Palmer, *Palmer's Law of Life*, 139.

Can you believe, given everything we know, that there are actually practicing chiropractors who don't do adjustments? I just want to shake these people. It makes me furious! Some people in recent years have even stopped using the word "adjustment." They have started calling chiropractic adjustments "manipulations" instead. Basically, they are caving to external pressure against chiropractic and the principle of correcting subluxations.[63] Many of them wouldn't dare use the word "subluxation," either. And they call themselves chiropractors!

You know what I want to say to these people? I want to tell them to just get the hell out of the profession. They're not doing anyone any favors.

Avoid the Mixers

> *"ADVICE to the sick who need [to] get well: Seek a chiropractor who adheres strictly to the single and simple Palmer's Law of Life, who confines what he does to that law. If he uses any medical method . . . he is NOT A CHIROPRACTOR AND IS NOT DELIVERING CHIROPRACTIC SERVICE."*[64]
>
> —B.J. Palmer

Chiropractors practice *chiropractic*. It's what we do, it's *all* we do, and the best way to do it is the same way we have been doing it since 1895. We don't do nutrition, physical therapy, massage therapy,

---

63 Williams, *The Meadowlands Experience*, 16.
64 Palmer, *Palmer's Law of Life*, 145.

acupuncture, etc. Those things have their place, but it is not in the chiropractor's office!

Nutrition is important, of course, so real chiropractors leave nutrition to trained nutritionists. Physical therapy can help people, so real chiropractors leave physical therapy to physical therapists. Massage therapy and acupuncture can be great, so real chiropractors.... Do you see where I'm going with this? If a chiropractor thinks you could benefit from any of these specialties, they should refer you to a specialist in that field. These people have a passion for what they do, too, and they're good at it. But *chiropractors* should not do these things.

> **Chiropractors who offer additional services beyond chiropractic care are what we call "mixers."**

Even chiropractic students are confused about this. I recently had a student ask me how to choose "what kind of chiropractic" he should do. As far as I know, there is only one kind of chiropractic. It's called straight, pure, principled **CHIROPRACTIC**. Principled chiropractic is all we need.

Here's what principled chiropractic looks like.

- The chiropractor lays the patient down on a table and checks their spine
- If the patient is subluxated, the chiropractor gives them an adjustment
- *That's it!*

More and more chiropractors are falling victim to the mixer mentality. It makes me angry to see all the extra crap some chiropractors do in their offices, all the additional services they offer, sometimes just so they can bill their patients more for care. . . . I'll tell you right now, that is **NOT** principled chiropractic!

These people who want to stretch, poke, laser, foot-bath, detox, cleanse—they're giving us all a bad name. The mission of chiropractic is to relieve nervous system pressure through specific adjustments. As soon as a chiropractor tries to add other services to their scope of practice, they are compromising and diluting the chiropractic principle. Our job is to deliver the goods, and the goods is the adjustment. *Nothing else!*

> *"Sick people go to a 'Chiropractor' (sign on the door) hoping he has some new principle and practice which will do what methods of medicine have failed to do. . . . If you see and get [the] same methods given by medical men— walk out, refuse to waste time and money."*[65]
>
> —B.J. Palmer

The most advanced care a chiropractor can provide is to simply adjust their patients with their bare hands. If your chiropractor is a mixer or tries to tack on additional services, my advice is to get out of there. Walk out the door and never go back.

The chiropractic principle is so straightforward, so fundamental, so simple, that many of us end up overcomplicating it.

Don't listen to the mixers. Listen to the principle!

---

[65] Palmer, *Palmer's Law of Life*, 28–29.

Look Within: Shed Your Husk

> *"It's very easy—you rise above the negativity to a higher plateau through LOVE, through dedication, through FAITH, through enthusiasm, through work, with programmed PLANNING, with the establishment of a definite, pre-planned major goal that you wish to accomplish in your life right now, this very week, this very minute. Don't take the easy road."*[66]
>
> —Dr. Sid Williams

Look in the mirror at your own eyes. Examine yourself. A lot of us are not where we want to be in life. We aren't even *who* we want to be. The solution: Shed the husk. Change yourself. It's as simple as that.

A husk can be anger. A husk can be jealousy, envy, a sense of mediocrity or uncertainty, or practically anything that prevents you from being the person you were meant to be. My hero, Dr. Sid Williams, used to say, "To become, act as if."[67] He used the bad habit of smoking as a classic example of a husk needing to be shed. "If you want to quit," he said, "don't say, 'I'm going to quit forever.' Start saying, 'I don't smoke.'"[68] Your problem(s) might be tougher than quitting smoking, but most husks are just habits that need to change.

The first time you try shedding your husk, it might not "take" right away. This happens to everyone, and I know it is discouraging. But if you keep at it—if you keep working, keep trying, keep showing

---

[66] Williams, *The Meadowlands Experience*, 7.
[67] Williams, *The Meadowlands Experience*, 60.
[68] Williams, *The Meadowlands Experience*, 94.

up—you are going to change. Every beautiful, detailed sculpture in every art museum around the world was once nothing but an ugly blob of clay or a hunk of shapeless, dirty old stone. But slowly, things were chipped away, and the beautiful details came into view. Every masterpiece begins hidden beneath layers of imperfect stuff that just needs to be chiseled away.

I don't want to mislead you; shedding husks is not fun. This is not a Tylenol experience. It does not happen quickly or painlessly. You won't start feeling the change until you start hurting first. When you persevere through that pain, you get the answers. You are able to show up, in the present, as the best possible version of yourself that is possible today.

> *"Bloom where you are."*[69]
>
> *—Dr. Sid Williams*

I was recently talking to a friend who was describing an experience mountain climbing. He was describing putting his fingers on the edge of the table, getting a grip in there, and pulling himself up by his fingertips wedged in this little crack.

Picture yourself in that situation: a hundred feet above the ground, holding on by your fingertips, with nothing but a tiny pin in the wall to (hopefully) hold your weight if you lose your grip and fall. You have no choice but to put your faith in your own strength and that tiny anchor. If you fall and that pin doesn't hold, you are dead.

As my friend described his experience up on the mountain, I found myself thinking that rock climbing is a lot like life. You give yourself an anchor—your purpose, your passion, your spouse, or your family—and you climb with the faith that it will hold you if you fall. At the end of the day, your own strength that will determine if you can propel yourself up to place the next anchor and get that much

---

[69] Williams, *The Meadowlands Experience*, 46.

closer to the top. And when you least expect it, life will open a crevasse beneath you that will give you one of those "oh shit" moments. It's all about how you choose to express yourself in those moments. Some people decide that this is the time to pack it up and go home. But really, those are the moments when you have to trust that whatever you've chosen to anchor yourself to is *secure*, and have the guts to pull yourself up!

Everybody falls. The only failure is when you fall and don't get back up. Failure is inevitable, but you don't have to be a loser. Take action and you can find solutions. Shed your husks until nothing is left but that strong person at your core who you always knew you should be.

The problem with life is that there is no top. You fight to climb, and you don't know when you'll be able to stop. It can seem overwhelming, insurmountable, because there is no end in sight, no end in mind, no place where you get to stop and rest. On the other hand, this is also a great thing because it defies us to create limitations. There is always room for growth.

The other problem is that too many of us are trying to make the climb with a lot of weight dragging us down. We are holding on by our fingertips with a bunch of extra baggage loaded on our shoulders. Whatever you think is holding *you* back, face it. Finish reading this section, put this damn book down, and go look at yourself right in the mirror and say, "I'm not letting this stuff hold me back anymore."

I used to put a glass of water on the back of the toilet before I left the house every morning. If I had a shitty thought during the day or something just wasn't right, I would visualize that thought or that thing going in the glass. Then when I came home at night, I would pour that glass of water down the toilet and flush it away. It created an action step for me. It helped me be more purposeful about the feelings holding me back.

Write Your Own Story

Sometimes, it is hard just to be a human. On certain days, the climb seems impossible, and when you think life can't possibly get any worse, it does.

A lot of us have lived through seriously tough times in our lives. I've been there, believe me, and it is no fun. All the pain, tragedy, heartache, mistakes, loss, and traumatic stuff that people have gone through in their lives—as children, as teenagers, as adults—some people call it baggage, but I call it what it is: shit.

Life is great, but it drags you through some *serious* shit.

Maybe right now, even as you're reading this, you are in the middle of some tough times—some shit. If you're not, times will *get* tough, I guarantee you that. Another disaster is always just around the corner, and no one is immune to that reality. Your shit is often a choice you made in the past. A failure or a mistake. I have slipped up a lot in my life. I admit that. If you're honest, I bet you could say the same thing about yourself.

The shit I've had to face made me who I am. It created me. Your shit—the unlucky breaks, the bad circumstances, and the lies you have carried around all your life—have all led you to create a "story" for yourself, and your story doesn't always serve you well.

A lot of people's stories read something like this: "If only *that thing* hadn't happened, then I could be happy." Or, "If only I hadn't screwed up so badly *that one time*, then things would be normal." But the most common story is simply, "Poor me."

You are always at risk of being sabotaged by your stories. You might be having a great day, but then you think about an old wound, and you immediately get nervous, irritable, or just plain depressed. Maybe you hear a song on the radio that makes you think of something or someone from your past, and suddenly, you are defeated. It seems like some people want to carry that crap on their shoulders forever. Here's my response:

Get over it.

> **God doesn't create victims; CIRCUMSTANCES create PERSPECTIVES that put STORIES in our brains.**

God chose you for a mission only you can fulfill. The shit you went through made you who you are. In some way or another, it prepared you for your mission. *You don't have time* to be sad or depressed or weak or defeated. As the poem goes, it is time to become "powerful beyond measure."[70]

There will be suffering. Stuff will happen, and it will happen when you least expect it. The question is, how will you handle it? You don't get to call a timeout when everything goes wrong. You still have to go to work and face your day, even when it's the worst day of your life. You cannot stop until it's time to take your last breath. And when you do take that last breath, you'll either smile because you're at peace with your life, or you'll cry because you'll know you could have done more.

I am willing to bet that you have some shit—something very heavy on your shoulders—preventing you from getting to the next level. You keep trying to change, but something keeps pulling you back. What is it? What is going on in your life? Think about it right now and cut it loose—throw it in the cup. See it flying into the cup. Each time you do that, it's gone. It's done! Flush.

This is not just a visualization exercise. It has real, tangible results. Once you recognize and acknowledge the negative stuff in your life and make a choice to actively rid yourself of it, it is no longer inside you. It becomes a memory. Your whole life is just memories, right? The weak life is the one that constantly stops and goes back to those

---

[70] Williamson, Marianne, *A Return to Love: Reflections on the Principles of "A Course in Miracles"* (New York: HarperCollins, 1992), Ch. 7, Section 3, 190.

memories and weak moments and fights them and fights them and fights them, until suddenly the clock runs out, and life is over. It's time to give that lifestyle up.

I am officially calling you out. What sort of shit are you carrying around that should have been dropped long ago? What is it you need to change? Look within and ask yourself, "Where am I weak, and why?" This can be tough, but it is necessary to the growth process. *Something* is holding you back.

Again, I urge you, put this book down for a minute, go look in the mirror, and ask yourself, "What is holding me back? How am I going to unshackle this weight and let myself grow?"

Chapter 9

Love and "Miracle" Stories

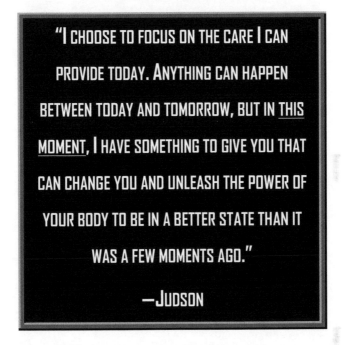

"I CHOOSE TO FOCUS ON THE CARE I CAN PROVIDE TODAY. ANYTHING CAN HAPPEN BETWEEN TODAY AND TOMORROW, BUT IN THIS MOMENT, I HAVE SOMETHING TO GIVE YOU THAT CAN CHANGE YOU AND UNLEASH THE POWER OF YOUR BODY TO BE IN A BETTER STATE THAN IT WAS A FEW MOMENTS AGO."

—JUDSON

People love to hear chiropractic stories. Things sometimes happen in the chiropractor's office that are pretty amazing—stuff that some people might even call "miracles." But I will be the first to tell you, they are not miracles.

Any miraculous-sounding story you've ever heard involved someone's atlas being adjusted.

How do I know this? Because when you adjust that tiny, circular bone at the top of the spine, it removes pressure on the brain stem, and when you remove pressure on the human brain, amazing things can happen. It's not a miracle. It is science. It is life.

The following is a story shared by Dr. Sid Williams in his book *The Meadowlands Experience*.

> "I used to talk all the time about a guy that couldn't see. . . . His mama brought him in for some care on his neck. I asked what was wrong with him. 'Well, he had a little accident, but he can't see out of his right eye.' I said, 'He can't see out of this eye? What's wrong with the eye?' 'The ophthalmologist says there's nothing wrong with it; he's just blind in that eye.' Three days after I adjusted him he brought his little New Testament in. He said, 'Watch, Dr. Sid,' and covered up his left eye and read that New Testament. His mother said, 'You performed a miracle.' I said I didn't; I just corrected the subluxation and cleared the interference in the nervous system that was causing that eye not to function."[71]

In the same book, Dr. Sid also discusses a woman diagnosed with multiple sclerosis. The doctors told her she would never walk again. She went to a chiropractor. Can you guess what the chiropractor found? A subluxation! The chiropractor adjusted the subluxation, and ten days later, she had no symptoms. Her diagnosis of M.S. was practically gone. The body had begun to heal itself. However, there was a twist to this woman's story. She stopped coming in.

Two months later, she came back with the same symptoms. The chiropractor adjusted her. Again, ten days later, the symptoms were gone. When she returned to her medical doctors with the news, do

---

[71] Williams, *The Meadowlands Experience*, 62–63.

you think they said, "Amazing! I'm sending all my patients to see a chiropractor!"? Of course not. They said, "Huh. Well, you must not have really had M.S., then."

If you talk to enough chiropractors, you will hear all kinds of stories of rapid transformations brought on by chiropractic care. Many people experience not only relief from symptoms but a reduction of symptoms associated with conditions like rheumatism, arrhythmia, asthma—everything from paralysis down to bedwetting and crossed eyes.[72] These are true stories, and they are not miracles. Subluxations are to blame. I will say it again: When you take pressure off the brain stem, the body heals itself.

Tommy's Story

I first met Tommy in 2012. He entered my office like a zombie—drooling, walking crooked, and barely speaking. He had hair down to his chest, a long, tangled beard, and was covered with tattoos. He looked like he hadn't showered in about sixteen years, and I'll be honest, he smelled like it, too.

It's easy to judge people who look a certain way, or to avoid people who seem "rough." But no one comes into the world like this. Things and events transform people, sometimes in traumatic, horrible, painful ways we could not possibly understand.

Tommy certainly had not been born that way. His story began one day when he was just a child, when he heard a gunshot in his home and ran downstairs to see what it was. His father had committed suicide. He had shot himself in the head, and Tommy was the one who found him. Imagine being a child and finding your own father like that.

---

[72] Williams, *The Meadowlands Experience*, 63.

If that wasn't bad enough, a couple of years later, Tommy found a second member of his family dead by their own hands. It was his younger brother. He had hung himself. If you have any brothers or sisters, close your eyes right now and try to imagine what it would be like to walk into a room and find them like that. I know it is a terrible image, but now imagine that the image never goes away no matter how hard you try—that you see it every time you close your eyes and relive it every time you fall asleep. Tommy pulled his little brother down off the noose to try to save his life. He performed CPR for a full hour until the paramedics arrived, but it was too late. His brother was dead, and Tommy would relive those events in his mind over and over again for years.

Tommy's life became a downward spiral of unfortunate events and self-destructive actions. He suffered from flashbacks, panic attacks, and nightmares. He experienced terrors and hallucinations in which things came after him that no one else could see. He was in and out of psychiatric hospitals, and doctors pumped him full of drugs. He tried to commit suicide to end the pain, but he failed. His diagnoses included but were not limited to bipolar disorder, schizophrenia, manic depression, and PTSD.

By the time he entered my office, he was a shadow of the person he had once been. He was nonverbal. He drooled. And I wasn't kidding about the smell. It was difficult to breathe while examining him; he was rotting from the inside out.

And do you know what I found during his examination? A misalignment in the upper cervical region. A subluxation.

It doesn't matter how "rough" somebody looks or how beyond hope they appear. The job of the principled chiropractor is to care for the person in front of us to the best of our ability, whatever their expression of life is right now. We do not judge about the past, and we do not make false promises about the future.

I choose to focus on the care I can provide today. Anything can happen between today and tomorrow, but in *this* moment, I have something to give you that can change you and unleash the power of your body to be in a better state than it was a few moments ago.

I found the location of the subluxation in Tommy's neck, and I adjusted him.

Tommy's mother continued to bring him in for regular care. During that time, I could see him getting progressively better, but as long as I live, I will never forget the moment his massive transformation became clear to me. He had been under care at our office for about three months when I turned the corner one day, saw him, and said, "Holy shit."

I realized that Tommy was walking straight. He had showered, he was talking, and he wasn't drooling. I live and own the principle of chiropractic, but even I was blown away as I thought back to the person who had entered my office three months prior. The kid who had been nonverbal and rotting from the inside out was now healing.

The reality hit me all at once—the reality that this thing called life is more powerful than I ever dared to imagine. Powerful beyond measure. Bigger than I could ever hope to understand.

***

Tommy's changes continued to astound us all. Until one day, I received a phone call. It was Tommy's mom calling to tell me he had been rushed to the hospital.

She went on to explain that some doctors had given him a flu shot. Every flu shot comes with a list of common side effects, including flu-like symptoms. Tommy had experienced some of those side effects, and they had led to some complications resulting in full-blown pneumonia. His mom wanted to know if I could come to the hospital to check him.

"Sure," I told her. "I have a full day at the office today, but tomorrow is my day off. I'll come in and see him then."

"It can't wait until tomorrow," she said. "They told me he's going to die."

I used my lunch break to drive to the hospital. Tommy's mom met me in the ICU and took me to his room. He was lying in a bed, unconscious. Tubes going in, tubes coming out, instruments monitoring his vital signs. He had been in a coma for eighteen days. Tommy's mom called me after they read him his last rites.

He looked more dead than alive, and the doctors had told his mother to prepare herself because he probably would not pull through this.

I couldn't help but feel pissed off. This young man—this human whose body had finally been given the chance to heal—was now holding on by a thread all because of a damn flu shot. For years, Tommy's doctors had attempted to treat his problems by pumping him full of drugs. Giving him a flu shot "just to be safe" was a continuation of that same old cycle. But this time, when they chose to stick that needle in his arm, they might have finally killed him. Maybe I don't blame them for trying. What else can you do with someone like that whose situation seems so hopeless?

You can adjust him. That's what you can do.

"They're wrong," I told his mom. "He's not gonna die."

She looked at me. "How do you know?"

"Because he still has life in him," I said. "This kid hasn't gone through all this crap just to die now. We're not gonna let him."

But adjusting Tommy that day would be easier said than done.

To fully appreciate the position I was in, you have to understand that the ICU is not a chiropractor-friendly environment. To be more precise, it is not an adjustment-friendly environment. There's nothing illegal about adjusting a consenting patient within a medical center, but hospitals are hypervigilant when it comes to any possible liability issues. If anyone had known who I was or what my intentions were that day, they would have been watching me like a hawk.

Doctors and nurses were constantly coming in and out of the room, and I knew if they saw me try to adjust Tommy, there would be trouble. They would probably call security and have me kicked out.

My only option—and Tommy's only hope—was for me to get in there, adjust him, and get out as quickly as I could.

If I had been too afraid to act or had decided to believe the opinions of the people diagnosing him, Tommy wouldn't have stood a chance.

When I saw an opening, I went in, and I adjusted him.

Tommy woke up immediately.

***

The next day, the phone rang.

"His numbers are changing," said Tommy's mom. "He's coming back! The doctors can't believe it!"

Of course they couldn't.

I was on my way to speak at Dynamic Essentials in Florida when I got the next call. This time, Tommy's mother was calling to tell me they had taken the tubes out of Tommy's throat, and he was breathing on his own.

Three days after I adjusted Tommy, he walked out of the hospital.

The doctors—surprise, surprise—couldn't believe it. But *why* can't they believe it? Why do people refuse to consider that there might be an answer beyond drugs? Why is it so hard to understand the power of a chiropractic adjustment? What are people afraid of?

When doctors are presented with a case like Tommy's, the last thing they want is to let someone touch him. To them, the safer option is to pump him full of drugs and leave him in a bed to see what happens. If Tommy's mother had told the nurses and doctors about what I had done, how do you think they would have reacted? With open-mindedness? With belief in the chiropractic way of life? I can tell you from experience, that rarely happens. More likely, they would have and been furious that I'd had the nerve to perform a chiropractic adjustment within *their* hospital, right under their noses, and they would have called the whole thing a fluke. But it's not a fluke. It happens all the time.

Tommy's story didn't end there. Not only did he fully recover from the pneumonia, but he continued to make huge strides forward. Tommy and I went through a lot together in the following years. I even started taking him to Dynamic Essentials and other chiropractic events and having him join me onstage during my talks. Anyone who has been going to Dynamic Essentials for a couple of years will remember him. It got to the point where I thought, *Why am I telling this story when I could let Tommy share it with people in his own words? If people think I'm full of shit, nothing I can say will change that, so why not let Tommy personally tell people what he's been through?*

Tommy shared his story with thousands of people and became a living, breathing demonstration of the transformative power of chiropractic care. A guy who had been nonverbal before chiropractic care was now onstage, speaking to the masses.

I am proud to have known Tommy, and I can't tell you how difficult it is for me to write these words, because at the time of this writing, Tommy recently passed away.

Unfortunately, it was the same old story. More well-meaning doctors gave Tommy some medication attempting to correct a minor health issue. Complications arose from the side effects of the medication, and this time, he died.

Dr. Sid Williams, the defender of chiropractic, had a saying: "Bloom where you are." It was not, "Bloom tomorrow," or, "Uproot yourself and move somewhere you can bloom." It was, "Bloom where you **ARE**." It's about today, right now, this very second, wherever you are in your life. That is what chiropractic is about. Allowing people to heal and become a better expression of life this very second, no matter what they have been through, who they are, or where they come from.

No one exemplified this philosophy better than Tommy. After a lifetime of pain, heartache, disease, drugs, and downright agonizing suffering, Tommy bloomed where he was. He became a different expression of life before our very eyes—a different human being. I feel blessed to have been allowed to see it happen. He's gone now, but he changed lives. Ask anybody who listened to him speak.

They'll remember Tommy. He was unforgettable.

Tommy was my friend, and I loved the guy. In the time I knew him, it was a privilege to watch him bloom—exactly where he was.

A Research Story

People hear my stories and either think they are amazing, or they think I'm lying. They want to see the research. You want research? I can introduce you to thousands of kids under chiropractic care, and we'll compare them to kids who are not getting adjusted regularly. The differences are staggering. You can see it in their expression of life.

I'm reminded of a young patient of mine. We'll call him Ben. Ben was an eight-year-old little boy with a single mom. He had been diagnosed with three different psychiatric disorders. At school, he had four aides who walked around with him all day long just to keep him in line, and he displayed such severe behavioral problems that his doctors had placed him on 911 alert. That means "one more strike, and you're out." If Ben acted up at home one more time, his mom would call 911, and the cops would come to take him away. The doctors basically considered him a lost cause and were ready to institutionalize him.

By chance or fate, Ben's mom ran into my wife Tammy. Tammy told her, "You need to get your son adjusted." Thankfully, she was receptive to the idea, and she brought him in. Ben was subluxated in the upper cervical region of his spine, so I adjusted him.

After Ben's first adjustment, the four aides who followed him around at school called home and asked his mom, "What happened to Ben? Something has changed. He's different."

By week three, Ben's life had done a 180 turn. He had been virtually uncontrollable when I first met him, but after just three weeks of chiropractic care, he would come in, look me in the eye, and shake my hand. He started getting smiley faces on his daily reports from school. The teachers couldn't believe it.

It was around this time that I received a call from one of Ben's doctors. The change in him was so evident that the doctors had asked his mom what was going on, and she had told them about the adjustments Ben was getting over at Judson Family Chiropractic.

Do you know what this doctor had called to tell me? "Dr. Judson, I don't agree with what you're doing over there."

He went on to basically accuse me of selling false hope and trying to cash in on a suffering family. This, from one of the doctors whose solution was to put an eight-year-old boy on 911 alert to be dragged away by the police and institutionalized indefinitely if he acted out one more time.

I have dealt with this sort of garbage in the past and can usually keep my cool, but this time around, the guy really rubbed me the wrong way. How much to do you think it costs to pay for multiple prescription medications for *the rest of your life*? How much do you think it costs to have someone institutionalized? We're talking about *millions* of dollars of "care" for a young kid with a single mom from a low-income neighborhood. And this doctor is accusing *me* of trying to make a buck? Who stands to gain more, here? And now that Ben was actually doing better, this doctor was calling me up not to express joy regarding his progress but to *confront* me about it.

Man, I wish I could have recorded that conversation. . . .

I said, "You son of a bitch. You don't agree with what *I'm* doing? You'd rather dope up an eight-year-old boy, take him away from his mom, lock him up in a psychiatric hospital, and steal his life away from him? I suggest you shut the fuck up, pal."

Ben's entire world changed because the pressure on his brain stem was released. How's that for research? The proof is in the results.

Love Your Kids

I was recently talking to someone about love. This guy was telling me about how he used to be a tough guy and is now trying to live in a space of love but doesn't really know how to do it. I told him, "Just start having kids."

Once you start having kids—when you hold your baby in your hands—this whole different side of you starts to open up. When you love something other than yourself to such a degree and realize that you have more love in you than you ever imagined, you learn how to love more. You even start to love yourself more.

As of this writing, my wife Tammy and I have five kids: Kylie (15), Sierra (13), Brooke (11), Kane (9), and Jaimee (5). People hear I have five kids and say, "*Five* kids? You're a little nuts!" It's really hard to have friends who don't understand what life is like with a high-volume family. You probably *do* need to be a little nuts. Everything is different. Just traveling with five kids is an adventure. All five of them are very athletic. They play a lot of soccer, basketball, lacrosse, and football. Plus, there have been competitive dance events, some modeling (Kylie was Miss Connecticut at one time, the two-time reigning champion), and all those sports and activities have us constantly on the move, sometimes driving to other states.

"Demanding" is the best word to describe life with five children. It ain't always easy! Balancing the responsibilities of being there for my kids, on top of the business, is sometimes pretty challenging, but as long as I stick to my routine and take care of myself and stay connected with wife Tammy, that's key. She has created that by making sure we are whole and connected and loving each other.

There are a lot of great times, and there are a lot of tough times. But I think the most important part of family life is just loving your kids, loving every minute with them, being present with them, having tough conversations, asking hard questions, and sometimes embarrassing them in front of their friends. . . .

I see my house as a boot camp for life. It's a place for all their friends to gather, and I'm the guy who asks them the hard questions. We talk to the girls about the hard things, right down to when they were going to their first dance. We asked them, "What will you do if a boy asks you to dance?" and we showed them what to do. We see it as our mission to prepare them. It's fun stuff.

All of my kids need attention. A lot of times, I just sit in a chair and I'm giving out hugs one after another. Then my son will throw a ball and bounce it off my head, so we go outside and play ball. Then I'll notice that one of my daughters needs a little extra attention, so I spend some extra time with her, which is a whole different energy.

Clear Since Birth

My kids have all been adjusted since birth, and every one of them is powerful and wild.

They're all athletes and students, just like any other kids, but they're fired up for life. And none of them have had a drug, pill, potion, or lotion in their bodies, because they haven't needed it. Because they are living clear.

When I tell people that my kids have never had a drug in them, they can't believe it. It's hard for people to understand this because of the society we live in. But these kids are living proof of the power of chiropractic.

Few children these days get to live the kind of healthy, clear lives my kids have. They don't understand why other kids are home sick—they don't know what that means. We had to have a discussion because they didn't understand what cough syrup was or how it was administered. They just looked at us and said how silly that was. "Just let the body heal. A cough is a good thing." That was a proud moment as a father, to realize, "Wow, these kids are really getting it!"

I see people at funerals, and I realize that the day will come when they're up there paying their respects to me—saying goodbye. I hope to leave behind multitudes who were impacted by what I did, but the greatest legacy I can leave behind is for my kids to say, "Dad did it the right way. He didn't sell out on the principle."

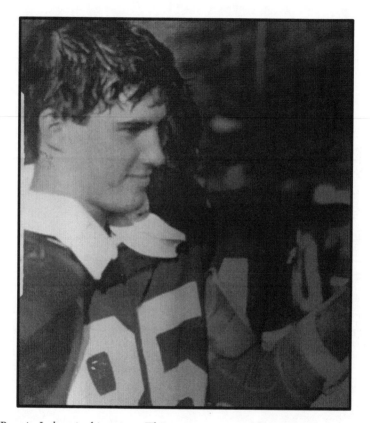

Ronnie Judson in his prime. This strong, young athlete pitched a no-hitter against Yale, was a brilliant student, and had everything going for him, until the day a massive subluxation in his upper cervical spine took it all way. A driving force behind my mission has been to share the truth of chiropractic around the world, so other families don't have to go through this same pain and tragedy. My mission was built on Ronnie's sacrifice—a sacrifice he did not choose.

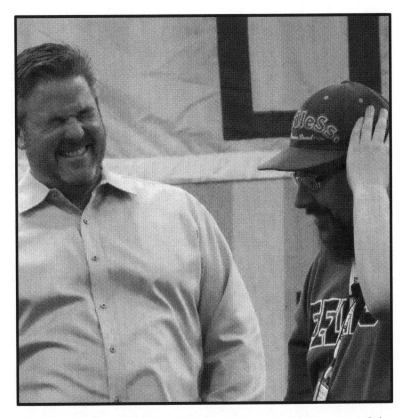

Sharing a laugh with Tommy at Dynamic Essentials. This was one of the many speaking events where I invited Tommy onstage to share his story in his own words. He was one of the most amazing people I have ever had the privilege to meet, and at the time of this writing, he has been gone for two years. As much as I was able to help him, he helped me in so many powerful ways. Love you, buddy.

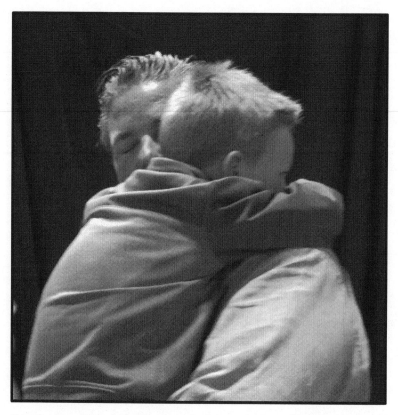

Pure healing. In an unloving world, love becomes the most powerful weapon we have. A bad heart can kill you. But a loving heart can change the world.

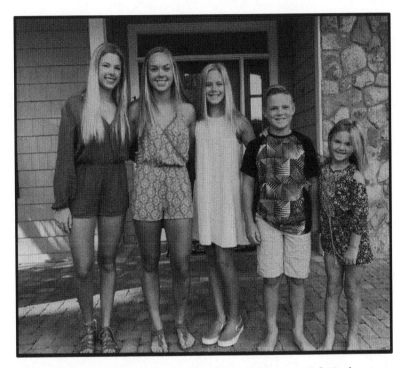

*The Judson team: Kylie, Sierra, Brooke, Kane, and Jaimee. Kids, I adore you.
You have taught me how to love beyond measure.*

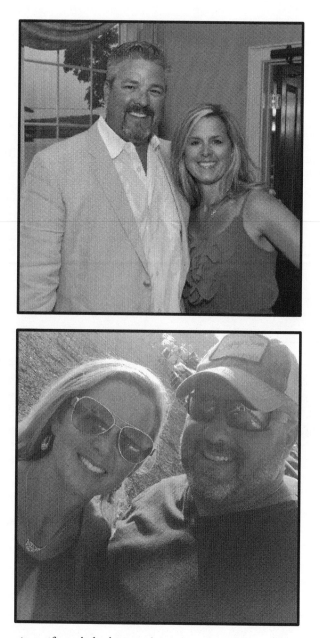

An amazing wife and the best mother I know. Tammy, thanks again for always being my rock, always standing by my side, and putting up with my craziness in my mission to make massive change in the world. I love you.

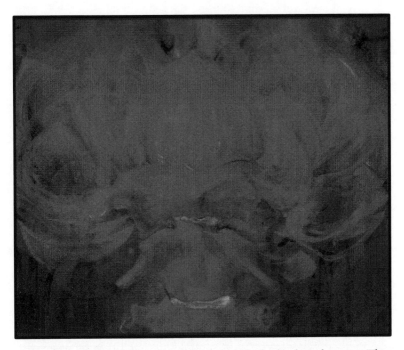

"Throughout time, the lotus has been a symbol of rebirth and purity. This remarkable flower emerges only by growing from the darkness of deep mud where it began its journey. It has been represented across many different cultures and by multiple religions.

"When I first met Dr. Steve, I was slightly skeptical and defiantly broken. I thought standing straight would always be painful, so I accepted that as a given. After a few weeks of being adjusted, I remember one day, something clicked. I was able to stand up straight without pain. He helped me not only by setting my posture straight, but also in becoming aligned. That has been an evolution of gaining understanding of unlocking my true potential in this life, and the work of Dr. Steve helps me to transform and blossom. This painting of the lotus, rising from the atlas, is a representation of that in my own life. I hope the message of my journey is able to resonate with those going through a journey on a similar path or anybody undergoing any journey.

"The darkness is all around us, and sometimes it may feel like it is within us. That's part of this painting—the journey from that darkness and how we're able to utilize it. How we're able to breathe life, to grow from it. Because just as the lotus, we must arise and be transformed. This is a life of transformation, and we have the ability to grow. This painting is a message of growth and a message of the clarity that we all have within us. It's about allowing your purest potential to come to light."

—Maria, painter, poet, and patient of Dr. Steve Judson

Chapter 10

Running from God

> "GOD IS GOOD.
>
> ALL THE TIME."
>
> —JUDSON

In August of 2009, Tammy and I put our house on the market. We were upgrading to a new place, designing and building a new home for our family. The real estate market was tough at the time. We knew our current house would take some time to sell, so we put it up for sale early so we would have plenty of time.

Imagine how we felt when it sold three days later!

At the time, we had four kids, and Tammy was twenty-eight weeks pregnant with our fifth child, a little girl. It was great that we sold the house so quickly, but it also left us with a small problem. The new house wasn't even close to being finished, but in order for the sale to go through, we had to move out of the old house right away. In the meantime, we moved in with my mother-in-law. (And just so you know, I have a great mother-in-law, so don't even think about feeling sorry for me.)

One night at my mother-in-law's, I had a nightmare. It started out as a normal dream. I was in an apartment visiting a man named Dick Hoyt.

Maybe you've heard of Dick Hoyt or his son Rick. Whenever I have patients who are feeling sorry for themselves or complaining about their lives, I tell them to go home and Google "Team Hoyt" for a change of perspective.

Iron Men

In 1962, Dick Hoyt and his wife Judy gave birth to a son, Rick. Rick Hoyt was diagnosed at birth with cerebral palsy and spastic quadriplegia. Dick and Judy knew from the time Rick was born that he would never learn to walk or speak. Those things were not a possibility for him. In Dick's own words, the doctors told them they should just "forget Rick" because he would be a vegetable for the rest of his life.

Forget their son. The doctors actually said that!

Dick and Judy wouldn't think of it. They refused to forget about their child or let him be put away in an institution. They took their baby boy home and did everything with Rick that you would do with a normal child. They spoke to him all the time and taught him numbers and letters. They weren't sure to what degree Rick understood them, but they kept at it.

As Rick grew older, he was unable to learn how to speak, but Dick and Judy could tell he was listening to them. They taught him basic vocabulary and moved on to more advanced stuff. When Rick was about ten years old, they raised some money and got a special computer system for him. Rick could communicate by highlighting letters on a screen and tapping his head against the device to spell words. They set up the computer, and everyone gathered around to hear what Rick's first words would be. But he didn't say "Hi Mom" or "Hi Dad" like everyone expected. The first thing he said was "Go Bruins." (The Hoyts are from Boston, and the Bruins were in the Stanley Cup that year.)

After that, Dick and Judy knew that Rick was not only intelligent but followed sports and rooted for his favorite team just like everyone else in the house. In fact, they learned that Rick loved athletics.

In 1977, when Rick was fifteen, he wanted to get involved in a benefit run for a local boy who had been paralyzed in an accident. Rick told his father he wanted to take part in the run. It was five miles long. Dick Hoyt had never competed in a single race in his life, but since Rick wanted to do it, Dick said he would push him in his wheelchair, and they would do the race together.

The day came, and Dick pushed Rick up to the starting line with the rest of the runners. Everyone thought it was a nice sentiment. A show of support. They figured Dick was just going to push Rick to the corner or something and that would be it. Instead, the run started, and Dick pushed his son through the entire race. All five miles. That night, after the race, Rick told Dick, "Dad, when I'm running, it feels like my disability disappears."

From then on, Dick and Rick competed in races every chance they got. Rick purchased a special running wheelchair, and Team Hoyt was born.

In 1981, Dick and Rick ran their first marathon, but that was only the beginning. Have you ever heard of the Ironman Competition? It's a triathlon: a 2.4-mile swim, followed by a 112-mile bike race, followed by a marathon (a 26-mile run), all done without a break between events. Team Hoyt rose to the challenge. For the swimming portion, Dick swam with a bungee cord attached to his waist, pulling Rick along behind him in a raft for 2.4 miles straight. When they got out of the water, Dick picked Rick up off the raft and placed him into a two-seater bike. Dick then pedaled for 112 miles. Let me say that again: 112 miles! When they got off the bike, Dick helped Rick into his running wheelchair and pushed him for twenty-six miles. Imagine doing all that, just to give your son the chance to do what makes him feel truly alive. This is not merely a symbolic gesture, either. There are mandatory cut-off times for Ironman events. You must complete each event within the cut-off time to move on to the next phase and finish the triathlon as an official Ironman. Strong, healthy, able-bodied men make it their life's goal to complete an Ironman Competition. Dick and Rick have completed it seven times.

At the time of this writing, over *fifty years* after they started, Team Hoyt is still competing. They have done over 1,000 races to date. Their motto is, "Yes you can."

Dick Hoyt, who had never even run a race before, dedicated his entire life to performing, literally carrying his son through life.

Rick Hoyt, who was born with the deck stacked against him, says if he woke up tomorrow without a disability, his first act would be to have his dad sit down in his wheelchair so *he* could push him.

Something's Not Right

You can see the spirit of devotion and love in this story, and that is why I tell my patients to look up Team Hoyt when things seem difficult. But that night at my mother-in-law's in December of 2009, I dreamed I was in an apartment in Boston visiting Dick Hoyt. In my dream, a little child ran across the room in front of us.

I looked at Dick. "Was that your son?" I said.

"No," said Dick.

At this point in the dream, Dick got up and left the room. Suddenly, three big guys came rushing into the apartment. They charged in, grabbed me, and pinned me down. One of them had a baseball bat. I struggled against them, but I couldn't move. I couldn't get away. They put the baseball bat to my throat and started choking me to death. I yelled, "Help! *Help!*"

I woke up screaming.

I rarely have nightmares, and I don't think I have *ever* woken up from a nightmare actually screaming like that. It was terrifying. Why was I talking to Dick Hoyt? Who were those guys? And who was that little child?

I sat up and realized it was four in the morning. I was in bed at my mother-in-law's house. Tammy, twenty-eight weeks pregnant, was awake beside me. She looked at me and said, "What's the matter? Is everything okay?"

"Yeah," I said. "Just had a nightmare, that's all."

Tammy said, "Everything's okay. Go back to sleep."

So I did.

What I didn't know at the time was that everybody had had a nightmare that night, including all of my daughters. When I woke up the next morning, Tammy was already awake.

"Steve," she said. "The baby. Something's not right."

That Face Doctors Make

You know, in my mind, I thought everything was probably fine. Maybe Tammy was just a little nauseous or something. Just one of those pregnancy things. Besides, we had been to the doctor a few days before, and everything looked perfect.

We decided to see our obstetrician just to be safe. Thankfully, the night before, one of my colleagues happened to text me asking if I needed any help at work tomorrow. At first, I said no. But then I decided, "Well, why not?" Since she was going to be at the office, I wouldn't have to worry about patients missing care because of my absence. Innate was working.

I went with Tammy to see our OB, but he was working at the hospital that day, so they sent us there. They admitted us and put us in a room to give Tammy an ultrasound.

Now, I want you to picture this. We are in our little room, and this female technician comes in. She's giving Tammy the ultrasound, running the scanner over her like usual, and watching the screen. We are just sitting there, waiting to hear what this lady has to say.

Then the technician pauses, and she makes a face.

She sits there making that face and looking at the screen, and she doesn't say anything. It feels like minutes go by, and I'm gritting my teeth, waiting for her to say something, thinking, *Lady, stop making that face and say something already.* But she just keeps staring at the screen.

Then she puts down the scanner, looks at Tammy, and walks out of the room. Doesn't say a word. Just leaves us there.

Tammy immediately puts her head down and starts crying.

"What's the matter?" I say.

"We lost the baby," she says.

***

For a while, no one comes in. We sit there alone in this quiet, little room with no word from anyone about what's going on. The minutes feel like hours.

Finally, a doctor walks in. He looks at each of us, adjusts his white coat, and sits down, leaning against the edge of the machine. He does the same thing the technician did: He just looks at Tammy, not saying anything. It's *that face* doctors give you. You know the one. Not good news.

At this point, I wanted to crack this guy in the jaw. After what felt like an eternity, he opened his mouth and told us that the ultrasound showed our daughter had died.

I don't even know how to describe what I was feeling in that moment. I couldn't believe it. It didn't make sense. We had *just* been to the doctor for a checkup, and everything was fine. I wanted to fight somebody. There was no way! How the hell did this happen?

"Okay," said the doctor. "We need to start you on Pitocin now."

"Pitocin?" I said. Pitocin is a drug used to induce labor. "What are you talking about? Why would she need that?"

He said, "Well, we need to deliver this baby now."

Basically, the doctor was telling me that we had not only lost our baby, but we had to go through the delivery process—today. Right now.

Tammy couldn't even go home. She had lost her daughter, and now she was stuck at the hospital and about to go through the worst physical pain a human being can endure. I can't even explain the hurt and anger I was feeling. I didn't want to fight somebody anymore—I wanted to kill somebody.

"Are you kidding me?" I said. "Can't you just knock her out and pull the baby out?"

I am sharing this with you for a very important reason. I know I was acting stupid, but if I didn't have such love in my life, I'm sure I would have done something *really* stupid. I wasn't even thinking anymore. Tammy kept me calm. I had to be present. It wasn't about me. My job was to be there for my wife. Still, I was furious.

Nothing made sense about this. People like to say things like, "Well, everything happens for a reason," or, "All things work toward good." I'm telling you, if someone had told me that at the time, I would have said, "Bullshit. Shut your damn mouth."

I was pissed at God. I was like, "Screw you, man. I'm becoming an atheist."

One of my good friends from the chiropractic organization Band of Brothers, Doug Stranko, came to the hospital and helped keep me calm. You want to talk about a real brother? He was there with us while Tammy went through labor. Doug's parents are pastors, so Tammy asked, "Doug, do you think your mom and dad could come out?"

Doug's parents came to the hospital, and my buddy stayed there with me the whole time. He even sat outside the room in the hallway while we delivered the baby. He and I didn't talk much through this whole experience; he was just there, which is all I needed.

We went through the labor process, and Tammy delivered the baby. The umbilical cord was wrapped around her neck. We were going to name her Lilly.

Doug and his parents came in and stood by our side. The nurses cleaned Lilly up and tried to hand her to me. They said I had to hold her because it was part of the healing process, to get closure, but I didn't want to. It hurt too much.

Finally, Tammy said, "You know what, Steve? It's okay. Go ahead." Then they handed me my baby.

So there I am, holding little Lilly in my arms. I'm looking at this tiny child, and she looks just like Brookie, our third daughter, and my heart is in pieces.

I thought about all those extra hours spent in the office. All the times I bent over backward to help patients and friends and family. All the people I touched through chiropractic—all the lives that were changed by my work. Yet I couldn't do anything for this one. I looked at her and said, "I'm sorry I couldn't help you. I've helped so many people, but I couldn't do anything for you. I'm so sorry." Standing there, holding my dead daughter, destroyed inside, all I could think was, *I have seen so many people saved. Why couldn't God save this one?*

Where are you now, God? Screw you, man. Just screw you.

As I handed Lilly to Tammy, I couldn't believe how calm my wife was. She was amazing. She *is* amazing. In fact, the doctor came in—he hadn't even shown up for the delivery—and Tammy said, "Hey, where were you?" He said, "Well, I'm fighting a cold and didn't want to be around you, so I waited." I was standing there thinking, *Screw him. Screw all of you.* But not Tammy. Right there, she started telling the doctor the story of chiropractic and telling him that he needed to get into our office and get adjusted. After all the shit she's just been through, she's basically putting on a patient orientation right here. The nurses were saying things like, "I knew I had to come in here because I haven't been feeling well." And Tammy was lighting them up, saying, "Well, you need to get into Steve's office and get adjusted!"

Meanwhile, I'm standing in the background with my mouth shut, just gritting my teeth. I couldn't say anything. I had to leave the room.

I called Tammy's mom to tell her what happened, and after I hung up, I just stood in the hallway crying. Then, lo and behold, one of my chiropractic patients comes walking up the hallway. What are the odds?

"Dr. Steve!" she says. "We just delivered our baby! Are you here delivering, too?"

"Yeah," I say. I'm wearing sunglasses, so thank God she can't tell I'm crying.

She says, "That's great! How's Tammy doing?"

"She's good," I say. "She's in there now."

"We just had a baby girl!" she says.

I say, "That's great. Good for you."

We hug. She introduces me to some people, and we talk a bit, all while I'm trying not to let her see what is going on in my mind.

I felt like I had died along with my daughter. I was done. I don't know how else to explain it. Just done. With everything. I decided, "I'm hanging it all up. I'm tired of taking care of everyone and serving and doing all this crap, and then I've got to hold my dead baby girl in the hospital."

Tammy was different. She's better than me. As we were leaving the hospital, she said, "I have a feeling this isn't the last time we'll be here."

The Flight Is Full

About a week and a half after this happened, my family was getting ready to go on a trip to Florida. Every year, right after Christmas, we would go away with some friends and their kids on vacation. Our families would spend a week together, and it was always a great time.

This year, with everything that had happened in our lives, we really needed it.

Everyone was excited for this trip. We woke up early the day after Christmas and rushed to the Hartford–Brainard Airport with an army of kids and all our bags loaded with stuff. The airport was mobbed with people, and after making it through all the normal hassles, we got to the counter to check in, only to discover that the airport did not have my name in their computer system. The rest of my family had tickets, but I didn't.

"Sorry," says the guy at the computer. "If your name's not on here, you're not allowed on the flight. It's full."

The thing is, I had a ticket. Tammy had all our receipts, our itinerary—everything that proved we had bought the tickets. But for some reason, mine wasn't showing up in their system. I asked if I could buy a ticket now to get on the flight.

"Nope, sorry," the guy said. "There aren't any tickets to be bought. I'm telling you, the flight is full, and everything else is booked. It's unlikely we'll get you on a plane before the end of the week."

"You had better hurry," another lady told Tammy and the kids. "The flight's about to leave."

I was ready to blow a gasket, but I stayed calm. I turned to my wife and said, "Tammy, go ahead. Take the kids and get on the flight. We'll figure everything out."

I said goodbye to my kids. I kissed my daughters. I hugged my wife. I told them I would figure it out and everything would be all right, and I sent them on their way. I watched them walk away, knowing that Tammy now had to take care of all four kids by herself, and my kids had to go on vacation without their dad.

As my family was just about to go around the corner, my little girl Kylie looked over her shoulder, and I could see that she was crying. There were tears running down her cheeks. Now, I was pissed.

I made sure my family was around the corner, and once they were out of sight, I let the guy have it. I started shouting at him, at the other people behind the counter—at pretty much anyone in sight. I was yelling. Screaming. I knew I was acting like an idiot, but I didn't care anymore. All my pain and heartache and frustrations came out at once.

Suddenly, I felt someone grab me by the shoulder from behind. Without even thinking, I raised my hand, turned around, and just slapped the guy.

It was a state trooper.

The state trooper was stunned. He stood there for a second, looking at me like I was nuts, and before he had a chance to say anything or pull out the cuffs, I yelled, "Do you know what my wife's been through in the last week and a half? And now, you people have to do *this* to her!"

And I told him. I told him everything that had happened. I told him about Lilly, what my wife had been through, and everything that had happened to us. And now, because these idiots had made a mistake, my wife and children were the ones paying for it. My kids couldn't even go on vacation with their dad.

The man had every right to arrest me. Instead, after hearing everything I had to say, he just nodded and said, "Okay, man."

The state trooper chatted privately with the people behind the counter. I don't know what he said or how it happened, but a couple minutes later, I was holding a ticket for a flight to Florida, scheduled to depart at 6:00 a.m. the next morning.

I was blessed to have gotten that ticket, but it didn't do much to change my mood. I got a little drunk that night, I have to admit. I was angry and off-purpose. It was a weak moment, and instead of going to bed, I went out, drank a bunch of beer, and just kind of felt sorry for myself.

I got to the airport early the next morning—I wasn't about to miss *this* flight—and went to get a cup of coffee to clear my head. I was still a bit drunk, still pissed off, feeling bad for myself, and seriously considering hanging it all up. I was ready to walk away from chiropractic and shut down the practice. It seemed like a fantastic idea at the time.

All those thoughts were still racing in my angry, stressed-out brain as I stood in line for coffee, when out of the corner of my eye, I noticed this guy coming up beside me. He stopped next to me, and I looked up and realized I recognized him.

Standing beside me, looking directly at me, was Dick Hoyt.

When We Are at Our Worst

I blinked. My jaw dropped. I couldn't believe it.

I said, "Wow...! Mr. Hoyt?" I was like a child.

I shook Dick's hand and introduced myself, but beyond that, I really couldn't tell you what I said to him—it's all kind of a blur. I know I didn't tell him about my dream. That would have been a little weird. And I know I didn't go into any detail about the stuff my family had been going through, but I did tell him I was a chiropractor and that I played videos of Team Hoyt in my office. I think I thanked him for everything he did, for just being him, and for the commitment he had demonstrated in his life. Or at least, it was something along those lines.

He was very polite about the whole thing. He said, "Wow, thank you. I really needed to hear that."

The whole experience was like an out-of-body experience. I didn't want to bother him anymore, so I turned and just sort of walked away, thinking, *Dick Hoyt lives in Boston. What are the odds he'd be in the Hartford–Brainard Airport at five-thirty in the morning, the morning after I missed my flight, a week and a half after the night my daughter died—and the same night I had a dream about him?*

I was about halfway down the airport terminal, thinking about all this, when I realized I had forgotten my coffee. I went back. Dick was still standing there, and he just looked at me and kind of smiled.

"I, uh, forgot my coffee," I said.

"Yeah, I know," he said.

As I walked away, I saw Dick's son Rick in his wheelchair with a bunch of people around him talking and asking questions. I looked at him, then looked back at Dick. Dick was watching me. I thought, *Oh, great. He probably thinks I'm some kind of freak stalker or something!* But Dick just smiled at me, and after a minute, the two of them left.

All I could do was stand there, dumbfounded. In that moment, something dropped on me. A weight was lifted off my chest. I can't quite explain it, but something suddenly hit me that said, without words, *Everything is okay.*

Before boarding the plane, I sent Tammy a text to let her know I was better and she didn't need to worry about me. I was all right. I got on my flight, put on my sunglasses, and cried just about the whole way to Florida. I took out some paper and wrote and wrote and wrote, bawling like a baby. To this day, I don't know what I wrote. I've never read it. But to me, this whole experience was God speaking to me.

As I sat on that plane, I felt His hand on my shoulder. It was like He was saying, "I've got your back, brother. You can stop mourning. It's okay. Lilly is okay, and you will be okay."

We like to say, "Everything happens for a reason," which I think is sometimes just a blanket statement to make us feel better or to avoid dealing with the reality of the shit we go through in life. I've been through a lot, but losing Lilly could have destroyed me. I really was ready to give up on everything. The experience could have curtailed everything I had worked for all my life. It could have killed me.

But the dream, the flight, meeting Dick Hoyt in person—God dropped in a whole series of events to keep me on-purpose in the middle of one of the toughest storms I've ever faced, proof to me that things really do happen for a reason, and He is there guiding us through it.

The passing of this little child made no sense to me. I was lost. But God had His hand on the situation the entire time, and the lesson I learned from it saved me.

In my mind, I was done having kids after losing Lilly. But fast-forward one year later, and I found out Tammy was pregnant—on Christmas Day! As far as the vacation I almost missed, I made it to Florida only a day late. I got to enjoy an awesome, relaxing time with my family. The air was cleared, so to speak, and everything was okay, because God told me so. God is good all the time, even when we are at our worst.

Chapter 11

Living On-Purpose

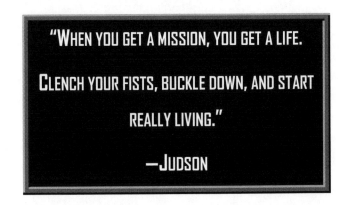

"WHEN YOU GET A MISSION, YOU GET A LIFE.

CLENCH YOUR FISTS, BUCKLE DOWN, AND START

REALLY LIVING."

—JUDSON

Not long after the events discussed in the previous chapter, Tammy and I were cleaning out the basement of our old house to prepare for the big move to our new place. In the basement, we found three pages from an old, yellow legal pad. As I skimmed over the pages, I realized it was a list I had made years before. I had written down one hundred goals, along with the dates when I was going to achieve them. Taking a closer look, I was struck by the fact that every single item had been achieved.

Just so we're clear, I'm not bringing this up to boast or to try to impress you. I am not bragging, and this is not a pride thing. I don't see it as an achievement, anyway. What I'm trying to show you is the power of living according to your purpose. It wasn't motivation or special talent that allowed me to achieve those one hundred goals. It was having a mission bigger than myself.

Know Your Mission

B.J. Palmer once wrote, "Most people are parasites living luxuriously on work produced by a handful of superior non-conformist minds."[73] Which of those two categories do you want to live in? I know which one I prefer.

You must have a mission on this Earth that is bigger than yourself—bigger than you ever imagined. Self-help author Napoleon Hill called it discovering your "definite, major purpose." I call it "living on-purpose."

Discover Your Purpose

Living on-purpose is a state of mind. It means living according to your mission and staying in tune with your "definite, major purpose" at all times. Reaching toward your ultimate goal in everything.

When you are on-purpose, you are keeping your mission in mind in everything you think, say, and do.

So, how do you discover this in yourself?

1. Ask yourself: What is my motivation? What is my vision? Where do I want to be five, ten, or twenty years from now? Write it down.

---

[73] Palmer, *Palmer's Law of Life*, 28.

2. Next, where are you right now? What does your life look like? More importantly, what do you want it to look like? What do you expect out of life? Write it down.

3. Finally, what is your purpose? What did God put you on this Earth to do? Look at yourself in the mirror and ask, "What's my mission in life? What is it I'm supposed to be doing that I'm not currently accomplishing?" Write it down.

I've said it three times, and I'll say it again: <u>Write this stuff down on paper!</u> I am serious about that part. Even if you never look at it again, the act of writing does something to your mind. There is something powerful about committing your thoughts and ambitions to paper.

Visualize yourself as the person you were meant to be, living according to your purpose.

If you don't know the answers to the questions I just covered, it is time for some self-examination. Too many of us just kind of coast through life from one thing to the next. You owe it to yourself to take the time to figure this stuff out. I don't have the answers for you. You must discover them for yourself.

If you have no passion, life is tough. I always hate it when I'm talking to a student and they say something like, "Well, I don't know what I'm supposed to do or where I'm supposed to go. . . ." I say, "Well, what do you want?" And they just give me a blank stare.

Kid, do yourself a favor and devote some serious time to figuring it out now, because if you don't, you might have to go through hell before you find it.

Think back to the rock climbing example. Everybody's mind is anchored to something. If you are not anchored to something positive, then you are anchored to something negative by default. For example, it used to be that everything I did was about proving myself to my parents, even though I didn't know that at the time. I now realize that if I live for someone else, I will fail.

You must find something that moves *you*. Something that digs up passion in you. When you have a mission—once you are conscious of your purpose—your life will never be wasted.

Your mission comes from within, but it also comes from beyond yourself. When you discover it, you will step into it and realize you're not *inventing* a dream; you're just accepting the mission that God had prepared for you all along. At times, it will be hard. You may need to change your thinking. You will need to add positive things to your life, and you may need to cut out some negative things. There will be certain people you just can't hang out with anymore—you know the ones I'm talking about. Leave them behind. They will sabotage your mission.

Muhammed Ali was once asked how many sit-ups he did during his workouts. His response was, "I only start counting when it starts hurting. That is when I start counting, because then it really counts."

You must be driven—when it counts.

When you are on-purpose, you do everything full-force, 110 percent. You work hard, and you train hard. You don't take "time off." Instead, you play hard and you rest hard! You're on-purpose all the time.

What's stopping you? Sometimes, it is a lack of vision. Other times, it is lack of commitment. Far more often, it is simply *fear*. There is no such thing as fear! We *create* it. So let's stop creating it and get to work!

Repeat after me:

I don't need to dwell on what's stopping me. I know what's stopping me, and I'm not okay with it anymore. I won't let it bind me. My life depends on it. Other people's lives depend on it. I don't need to change. I am changed.

When you get a mission, you get a life. Most of us are not currently accomplishing ours. If you're not, it is time to start working toward it. And if you are, then your mission needs to get *bigger*. Clench your fists, buckle down, and start really living.

Time

Dr. John Boutwell at Dynamic Essential always says, "The cemetery is full of people who didn't have time."

Time is the most valuable commodity in existence—the most precious gift we are given. Love can be found, lost, and found again. Money can be gained, wasted, and regained again. Weight can be gained and lost . . . and it can certainly be gained right back again if you're not careful.

But time can only be lost. Whether you waste it or use it well, either way, it is gone. You never get it back. Minutes tick away and disappear forever. And when your time is up, that's all she wrote.

We don't all get the same number of days, but we all get the same number of hours in a day. The question is, how will you use that time?

Your life is ticking. It's you versus you. Let's make it happen!

"Now, what I want to do is help you and guide you toward knowing what a real, major purpose is. . . . I want us to begin to learn how to direct our attention so that we can look more at the stream and less at the leaves that float in the stream. Now most people are spending the majority of their lives concentrating on the leaves, and those leaves—those small things—are difficult to turn loose in many instances, because they at least offer some security. But the big ones—the seers, the saints, the lovers, the people with the big ideas, the people with space, the people with capability—know how to watch, feel, and experience the stream. And in experiencing it, it continually opens them up for receptivity. It keeps their minds stimulated at a higher vibration, so they can deal with the innate consciousness within, so they are able to overcome obstacles, overcome temporary defeat, overcome temporary setbacks, learn how to face disaster, learn how to face tragedy, learn how to face worry and fear and regret without giving them anything, without giving them any attention, without giving them any awareness."[74]

—Dr. Sid Williams

---

[74] Williams, *The Meadowlands Experience*, 4–5.

Purpose and Peace

Peace is a huge goal in many people's lives. If you have a vision and a purpose, that is peace!

Odds are, you have gotten hurt and beaten up over the course of your life—deceived, betrayed, and wounded. You should know by now you weren't meant to carry that burden around forever. Your job is to heal from it, whatever it was. If you don't, peace will always be beyond your reach.

God made you who you are, and he made you divine and perfect. Does He place us on this earth just to go through the motions? Or does He pick every one of us to excel at something, to help each other, and to change the lives of others? I know what I believe. How about you?

Sometimes, bad things happen. God doesn't always answer our prayers. We must accept that. We must walk by faith, not by sight. Consider my story in the previous chapter, or Ronnie's story. Even when stuff happens that seems tragic, God will align events and people and feelings to help pull you through it. If you listen to Him, He will help you stay on-mission and on-purpose, even in your darkest times. Sometimes, you will meet someone who impacts your life profoundly, and you'll never see them again. Other times, a person sticks around who you never expected to affect you at all and becomes a major influence on your life, always pushing you forward. When you put it all together, it's unbelievable.

I always tell people it's good to pray, but don't wake up every day asking God for stuff. Just say, "God, what can *I* do today to love and serve more? What can I do today to give people a message that will help them change their lives?" Now that is peace!

Develop a System

People spend their whole lives trying to find the magical combination that will prevent bad things from happening to them. It's wasted effort! The only real solution is to have a system in place to deal with the bad stuff when it hits. A disaster plan. A plan that answers the question, "Okay, what am I going to do when times get tough?" Not if, but when.

I have plenty of shitty days when my former self threatens to return. It happens to all of us. When those things creep up, I have systems in place to pull me back and anchor me. Personally, I use my family. I use my faith. I use pictures, music, and positive YouTube videos. These things help redirect me and keep me on course. It helps me keep facing my shit head-on and developing myself amid the storms.

When you start living a purposed life from a state of abundance, it is like a door opens inside you. The trick is to never let anybody shut that door, no matter the circumstances.

Developing and using your recovery system is a divine art. You must look within your soul and know your door will never shut. You will never go back to the person you used to be, no matter what life throws at you.

The Shit Is Never Far from the Fan

There's a story about a woman who brought her child to Gandhi. She says to Gandhi, "My son eats too much sugar. Can you tell him to stop?" Gandhi looks at her and says, "Bring him back in a month." She says, "A month?" He says, "Yes. A month." So this woman leaves, waits a month, and comes back. Gandhi looks at the child and says, "Stop eating sugar." The mom's response is, "Couldn't you have told him that a month ago?" Gandhi says, "No, I couldn't. I hadn't stopped eating sugar yet."

Your words and your beliefs must be congruent with your lifestyle. You have to "walk the walk." If you are incongruent in any area of your life, it will show up when the pressure is on—when you have to make a sacrifice or when the shit hits the fan. (And believe me, the shit is never far from the fan.)

Many things happen that we cannot control. Situations in life will try to crush your spirit. Push through and tell yourself, "It's gonna be okay." I always say, "Jesus went through a hell of a lot worse." From that perspective, our shit is nothing.

Face it head-on. Deal with it. Embrace it, own it, and make it part of who you are because it never goes away. You can keep carrying it, but instead of letting it weigh you down, wear it like a badge of honor! If we let it control us, it will eat away at our minds and souls.

Toxic Living

When most people think of being in a "toxic" state, they think of it as something physical like a poison. But destructive thoughts like fear, anger, and depression can do just as much to create a toxic state in your body as any poisonous substance. If this describes your daily mindset, do <u>whatever it takes</u> to change those feelings. Your emotions and your state of mind can literally kill you.

When you don't like the way your hair looks, you get a haircut, right? Well, if you want to save your own life and escape the toxicity, I suggest you apply the same thought process to whatever creates negative emotions in your mind. If you don't like it, cut it. Maybe for you that means unplugging something and throwing it away; calling somebody up and reconciling; giving someone a hug; telling someone you love them, or just looking in the mirror and saying "I forgive you." Maybe you need to do the glass of water exercise from Chapter Eight. Whatever works for you, do it. Clean up your life.

> *Many of you are sitting in the office, negative about your friend that's doing better than you are, mad at your wife, mad at your mother-in-law, mad at the bill collectors . . . mad at everything, just thinking about it all day long. . . . Your emotions have been built up by reacting to fear and frustration, and you're being driven by this constant chatter inside your head.[75]*
>
> *—Dr. Sid Williams*

Ask for help if you need it. Ask the questions you don't want to ask because they make you feel embarrassed. Go on and embarrass

---

[75] Williams, *The Meadowlands Experience*, 44–45.

yourself if you have to! Your life is at stake. A little embarrassment is worth it.

Your personal demons might not be fears. They might be anger or envy or self-doubt. Determine what is holding you back. That is the first step toward learning how to overcome it. You won't have to spend your days dwelling on negative emotions anymore. Instead, you can better invest your time by focusing on the mission God sent you here to accomplish. There is nothing left to do but show up and deliver the goods.

Wouldn't it be nice to be free to do that? To just get on with your life and do what you were called to do?

To reach this point takes vulnerability and exposure. No one likes it when other people can see their baggage. When you reach that point, and the worst parts of you are on display, you will have two choices: You can clean it up and get better, or you can run away.

Many people would rather hide. It is the more comfortable in the short-term. It's like a drug addict at an intervention. Those who aren't ready or willing to change will react negatively. They will try to hide the truth, and they may become furious at you for exposing this part of them. But when an addict wants to change, he won't try to hide from reality. He will own up to it and work toward a new reality.

Be prepared. When your baggage is exposed, people might judge you for it or call you out. If they are humble—if they're sharing constructive criticism and challenging you to change yourself for the better—then they are probably worth listening to.

You do not have to be perfect. No one is. But I want you to understand that you don't have to carry all this shit around with you anymore. It is preventing you from expressing your potential. That's why people feel like their lives are so stifling. That is why it's so hard to break through.

Your shit is not only slowing you down from accomplishing your mission—it's *killing you*! Time to get rid of it forever.

Chapter 12

The Genius of Living Innately

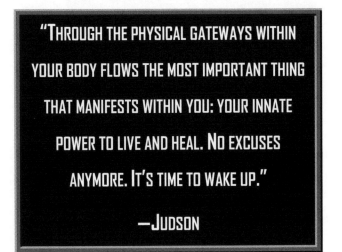

"THROUGH THE PHYSICAL GATEWAYS WITHIN YOUR BODY FLOWS THE MOST IMPORTANT THING THAT MANIFESTS WITHIN YOU: YOUR INNATE POWER TO LIVE AND HEAL. NO EXCUSES ANYMORE. IT'S TIME TO WAKE UP."

—JUDSON

As mentioned previously in this book, I am often asked to speak at chiropractic and health-related events. That means on top of running Judson Family Chiropractic, I am also frequently traveling all over the country to spread the message of principled chiropractic. On any given weekend, I might be speaking to a room of hundreds or thousands of people or broadcasting the truth to millions around the world. As a result, many people are surprised—and a little horrified—to learn that I usually step onstage with nothing prepared for my audience. I go out there with literally no idea what I'm going to talk about.

This isn't because I am a poor planner or because I am naturally spontaneous or something. It is a strategy. And I definitely don't see it as being unprepared. It's the best preparation there is! I allow myself to go where I am led. To me, that's what it means to follow the road of innate intelligence.

> *"Over and above, back and in behind ALL power and its expressions in a body, is 'that something' which no man has ever seen, felt, tasted, heard, or directly sensed—that GREAT UNKNOWN SOURCE—the Universal Intelligence and its fragment of the whole in units—Innate Intelligence."*[76]
>
> *—B.J. Palmer*

As discussed earlier, innate intelligence is the set of instructions your brain sends to your body to tell it how to operate. When you are free of subluxations (free of interference), your body is able to receive and carry out these instructions to the letter.

But there is another side to innate intelligence. When you are truly *clear*, operating in your daily life with no interference and getting checked regularly to make sure your atlas is perfect, those instructions will sometimes hit you in remarkable, unbelievable ways.

Instead of overthinking things, you find yourself acting intuitively. Instead of wondering about something, you will have a sense that you just *know*. In a way, these instructions are doing more than telling your body how to function; they are teaching you how to live your life.

> *"Innate reaches out over into the finite mind of [the] educated man, in what education crudely calls intuitions, hunches, instincts, inspirations, which we prefer to call 'thought flashes' from Innate, which sneak up on our educated blind side, slip in what they want you to know or do,*

[76] Palmer, *Palmer's Law of Life*, 13.

which they hope you will accept, grasp, heed, and do. They come as 'thought flash' ideas, desires, intentions, from a source above and beyond you to help and encourage you to be greater than education realizes.[77]

—B.J. Palmer

I live innately in, well, just about everything I do. The principle of chiropractic totally envelops my life. I am constantly plugged into that "**GREAT UNKNOWN SOURCE**" B.J. Palmer talked about. Every day, I am listening to innate's "thought flashes"—those little urgings that suddenly enter your mind as if out of nowhere—because I have learned that they *don't* come out of nowhere! There is a reason these things pop into your mind. Listening to innate is like being tuned in to a radio station that never goes out. The more you listen to it, the louder it gets. And when you listen and obey, that is called living innately.

Have you ever had a conversation with someone, and it takes over your thoughts and feelings for the rest of the day? Or the rest of the week? Maybe it was a positive conversation, or maybe it was negative. Maybe it even hurt your feelings a little, or it felt like the person was stepping on your toes in some way, calling you out on something. Either way, days go by, and you still just can't stop thinking about that conversation for some reason. Weeks or months later, something happens, and you suddenly realize the message you were supposed to learn from that encounter. It's no accident when that happens. Innate sends these things your way. It's how we grow. Living innately is simply accepting that reality.

Now, here is the amazing part. Chiropractic care allows you to be more in tune with innate.

---

[77] Palmer, *Palmer's Law of Life*, 23.

At first, it will be flashes of thoughts that seem to come from nowhere, helping you in times of trouble. Helping you put out the fires in your life. But eventually, the day will come when it's not about putting out fires anymore. Innate intelligence will be actively guiding you down a path to create such abundance in your life that it's like, my God, there is nothing to be worried about! Nothing to be angry about! Nothing to be sad about!

People ask me, "How will I know I am hearing the voice of innate?" It takes a lot of work. It takes work to get clear. It takes work to shed your husk (or husks). But eventually, you won't have to *try* to listen to innate anymore; it just comes through you automatically.

"'Genius,' as we dub it, is nothing more or less than the individual who listens, accepts without question and permits development of a superior knowledge FROM WITHIN to flow freely without questioning that which flows freely from above-down within-out—that's why genius is genius.

He has learned to respect those subterranean thought flashes, thereby keeping pathways open and receptive. If he wakes in the night with 'an idea,' he captures it then and there, doing the thing, whatever it is, when it is coming. Most would roll over and go back to sleep and forget it. Genius is genius because they have and utilize that peculiar faculty of absorbing from a source greater than they know, the inherent capacities of receiving and using those 'inspirations, aspirations and perspirations' that

> *come so freely from within out, refusing to reject from within-out."*[78]
>
> *—B.J. Palmer*

There is also a second part to living innately. It occurs when you become the message-sender instead of the message-receiver. When you suddenly get a feeling, an urge, or a "thought flash" out of nowhere that tells you to say something to someone, or to call someone up who you haven't thought about in a while, or just to hug someone for no reason.

There is a message in everything you think, say, or do. Innate never stops giving you signs and signals. It's the most powerful gift God has given us to express ourselves in life. You just have to listen to it. When you are connected and aware and present to pick up on the messages, your life is awesome.

Our Far-Reaching Thoughts and Actions

We all get hurt. We are hurt by our parents and our friends. Some of us are hurt by our spouses, our children, our coworkers, our churches. . . . We are hurting.

When people I know and care about are hurting, I tell them, "It's okay, but you have to have faith." You will always be okay when you are connected to the source. Even when tragedy strikes, innate leaves messages around you reminding you that everything is okay.

We like to believe everything happens for a reason, but sometimes I think we mistakenly get the impression that all our hurt occurs so that *we* can learn a lesson from it or benefit somehow down the road. In reality, we are sometimes given the responsibility of going through

---

[78] Palmer, *Palmer's Law of Life*, 34.

some sort of pain so that someone else—maybe someone we'll never even meet—can receive a message.

Everybody in life is called upon to make sacrifices that will serve as lessons for someone else. When you come to terms with that reality, you can be at peace with the problems that get thrown your way. All the personal disasters that make you say "Why me?" will start to make sense. You will start to realize, "Maybe I'm going through this because somebody else is supposed to learn a lesson from it." With this in mind, you will be able to keep moving forward. Everything you think, say, or do will in some way directly affect your life or the life of someone else.

Here's something you can try today. Just walk up to a stranger and say, "Hey, how're you doing? It's good to see you!" And hug them. Chances are they will be pretty confused. They might hug you back just to be polite. Maybe they'll smile a little and think you've mistaken them for someone else. Don't even strike up a conversation. Just hug them and walk away. It will be awkward, but I think innate wants you to do it. I guarantee that person will think about you for the rest of the day—or the week! Maybe they will go home and tell their family about the weird person who hugged them. Or maybe they will feel abundant gratitude in their hearts because they really needed that today. Maybe your simple act will help heal them of an old wound or even save their life. Maybe you will be delivering a message to someone who was hurting badly and desperately needed it.

"I Can't See a Chiropractor Because. . . ."

There are always plenty of reasons not to take a great opportunity, but when it comes to reasons people "can't" see the chiropractor, I have heard them all. They are all bullshit excuses, and if these people knew the truth, their thinking would change really quickly. In my experience, the excuses pretty much boil down to one of two things.

1. I don't have the **TIME**.
2. I don't have the **MONEY**.

Many people say they don't have the time to go to the chiropractor, but if you ask me, *time* is exactly what is at stake. While I can't guarantee that you will live longer if you're under chiropractic care, I *can* guarantee that diligent care for your spine, brain stem, and central nervous system will vastly improve the quality of the time you do have. I can say with 100 percent certainty that when you are under regular chiropractic care, you are in a better overall state, mentally and physically, than someone who neglects their spine, brain stem, and central nervous system. It's basic logic. Take better care of the system, and it will take better care of you.

For those who say they don't have the *money*, here is my response to that age-old excuse: Many of my patients report that they spend less money per year since getting under chiropractic care than they used to spend at the family medical doctor's office buying antibiotics, flu shots, and painkillers. Don't even get me started on the financial cost of living with subluxations when all these "common problems" steadily become compounded into major health issues that bleed your bank account dry. Chiropractic care changes all that.

Having read this book, you can no longer claim ignorance. You know the truth. I invite you to step above the B.S. excuses and discover your new, awesome life. Refuse to waste your *time* in the waiting room at your family medical doctor's office; refuse to waste your *money* on drugs.

> *"The Innate man, hard to satisfy, moves forward. Educated man, satisfied with what he has done, moves backward."*[79]
>
> —B.J. Palmer

How to Find a Principled Chiropractor

In 2002, some of my colleagues and I started a group called Band of Brothers, a community of principled chiropractors devoted to serving people, connecting, holding one another accountable, and being a support system for chiropractors around the world. We also serve as a resource for anyone trying to find a principled chiropractor in their area to help them. The following are some of our beliefs.

- *We believe the* **POWER** *that made the body* **HEALS** *the body. It happens no other way.*

- *We believe that there is a Universal Intelligence is in all matter and continually gives to it all its properties and actions, thus maintaining it in existence. The expression of this Intelligence through matter is called Innate Intelligence and* **IS** *the Chiropractic meaning of Life. A vertebral subluxation causes interference with the transmission of Innate Intelligence, which leads to incoordination and dis-ease. Through a specific, scientific Chiropractic Adjustment, the subluxation is corrected, and health, vitality, desire, and coordination are restored.*

- *We believe many chiropractors are lost, and it is our obligation to show doctors, both young and old, that* **PRINCIPLED** *Chiropractic*

---

79 Palmer, *Palmer's Law of Life*, 25.

will allow our community, state, nation, and world not only to survive, but thrive.

- *We believe we are called into service to serve humanity through the practical application of the science and Chiropractic, the dominion over the Philosophy of Chiropractic and the mastery of the art of the Chiropractic Adjustment.*

- *We believe every Chiropractor should have an awakening to the Dynamic Essential—the "New Spirit" born into the consciousness after people become aware, humble, and obedient to the will of God within themselves.*

To find a principled chiropractor, visit the Band of Brothers website: www.chiropracticbandofbrothers.com. We have a tool that allows you to search for principled chiropractors registered with us. You can also contact someone directly in Band of Brothers who may be able to recommend a principled family chiropractor in your area.

Wake Up!

> *"We never know how far-reaching some thing we may think, say or do today will affect the lives of millions tomorrow. It is better to light one candle than to curse the darkness."*[80]
>
> —B.J. Palmer

YOUR BODY CAN HEAL ITSELF.

How amazing is that statement when you really think about it? It is truly awesome! Say it out loud: "My body can heal itself." Close

---

[80] Palmer, *Palmer's Law of Life*, 8.

your eyes and say it again. Meditate on the power of that incredible truth.

Personally, I started out on my life's journey thinking I was just another guy. Just some dude from New York. Nothing special. Even after I had accepted the call to chiropractic, I never could have anticipated where it would lead me or the responsibilities that would be entrusted to me as a result. But I have come to realize that it is my God-given mission to take this thing to the next level. To a level that no one has ever reached before. To not only serve the people in my community through chiropractic care but to educate the public, fuel the fire, and spread this message to the masses.

I am only now starting to understand that God has far bigger plans my life than I ever dreamed of. It is my mission to wake up humans.

At the core of that mission is the story of Ronnie Judson, and how a single moment on a football field in Pennsylvania changed the course of a young man's life, along with the lives of his entire family. Too many people like my brother have had their lives stolen from them. The passion within me is to help people like Ronnie—and families like mine—learn the truth so that they can avoid long-lasting physical and mental pain and dis-ease.

This mission is about restoring health, ease, and vitality to human beings. It is about helping people find hope and love for one another, and compassion and faith within themselves. To help people realize that their lives can be better if they follow certain principles and take massive action to be better human beings. To be more connected to the source, and more loving and nurturing to each other. You achieve this by making a conscious effort to stay clear—to get your atlas checked and to care for your central nervous system.

Through the physical gateways within your body flows the most important thing that manifests within you: your innate power to live and heal.

No excuses anymore. It's time to wake up.

I see books all the time, advertising "the ten steps" for this or that, or the "five steps" to success, or the "seven steps" to health. Everyone wants to believe that the secrets to health, success, and happiness can be distilled down to a few easy steps. The truth is, it's even simpler than that. Multiple steps would only overcomplicate this message. Here is the real secret.

The One and Only Step to Health

1. **Get your atlas checked**

Get clear. Discover what it means to live the healthy, fulfilling, abundant life you were always meant to live.

It is time to bloom where you are, discover your purpose, and start spreading this word to others. If you know someone who needs to hear this message, send them a copy of this book, or send them to www.judsonchiropractic.com/wakeuphumans for a free educational resource that could change their life.

Let's change this world. Let's wake up humans.

Appendix

Chiropractic Resources

www.chiropracticbandofbrothers.com
www.judsonchiropractic.com/judson-101
www.facebook.com/judsonchiro
Instagram @drstevejudson

Stephenson's Thirty-Three Chiropractic Principles

1. THE MAJOR PREMISE
   a. Universal Intelligence is in all matter and continually gives to it all its properties and actions.
      i. *"Life is a combination of intelligence, force, and matter. Matter makes up the material universe—intelligence is the immaterial universe, and force is what binds them together."*[81]

2. THE CHIROPRACTIC MEANING OF LIFE
   a. The expression of intelligence through matter is the Chiropractic meaning of life.[82]

3. THE UNION OF INTELLIGENCE AND MATTER
   a. Life is necessarily the union of intelligence and matter.
      i. *"Without intelligence, matter could not even exist. Without matter, intelligence could not be expressed."*

---

[81] Stephenson, *Chiropractic Textbook*, 236–237.
[82] Stephenson, *Chiropractic Textbook*, 237.

ii. *"The study of physics shows us that some form of energy gets into matter to make it move. Without this energy, matter is inert."*[83]

4. THE TRIUNITY OF LIFE

a. Life is a Triunity of having three necessary united factors; viz., intelligence, force, and matter.

5. THE PERFECTION OF THE TRIUNITY

a. In order to have one hundred per cent life, there must be one hundred per cent of intelligence, one hundred per cent of force, one hundred per cent of matter.

i. *"The expression of intelligence may be hindered by the limitations of matter."*[84]

6. THE PRINCIPLE OF TIME

a. There is no process which does not require time.

i. *"Force is a word implying action; action is a process. Action implies one event after another. One even after another, forming a series, implies time."*[85]

7. THE AMOUNT OF INTELLIGENCE IN MATTER

a. The amount of intelligence for any given unit of matter is always one hundred per cent, and is always proportional to its requirements.

i. *"No power less than the Creator could deprive a unit of matter of its share of intelligence; but the limitations of matter may prevent the expression of that intelligence."*[86]

8. THE FUNCTION OF INTELLIGENCE

a. The Function of Intelligence is to create force.

9. THE AMOUNT OF FORCE CREATED BY INTELLIGENCE[87]

---

[83] Stephenson, *Chiropractic Textbook*, 238.
[84] Stephenson, *Chiropractic Textbook*, 239.
[85] Stephenson, *Chiropractic Textbook*, 239–240.
[86] Stephenson, *Chiropractic Textbook*, 240.
[87] Stephenson, *Chiropractic Textbook*, 250.

a. The Amount of Force Created by Intelligence is always one hundred per cent.

10. THE FUNCTION OF FORCE[88]

   a. The Function of Force is to unite intelligence and matter.

11. THE CHARACTER OF UNIVERSAL FORCES[89]

   a. The forces of Universal Intelligence are manifested as physical laws; are unswerving and unadapted and have no solicitude for structures of matter.

12. INTERFERENCE WITH TRANSMISSION OF UNIVERSAL FORCE

   a. There can be interference with the transmission of universal forces.

13. THE FUNCTION OF MATTER

   a. The Function of Matter is to express force.

14. UNIVERSAL LIFE IN ALL MATTER

   a. Force is manifested by motion in matter; all matter has motion, therefore there is universal life in all matter.

15. THERE CAN BE NO MOTION IN MATTER WITHOUT THE EFFORT OF FORCE

   a. Matter can have no motion without the application of force by intelligence.

16. UNIVERSAL FORCE IN ALL KINDS OF MATTER

   a. Universal Intelligence gives force to both organic and inorganic matter.

17. CAUSE AND EFFECT[90]

   a. Every Effect has a Cause, and every Cause has Effects.

      i. *"The study of Chiropractic is largely a study of the relations between Cause and Effect, and Effect and Cause."*[91]

---

[88] Stephenson, *Chiropractic Textbook*, 250.
[89] Stephenson, *Chiropractic Textbook*, 251.
[90] Stephenson, *Chiropractic Textbook*, 256.
[91] Stephenson, *Chiropractic Textbook*, 256.

18. THE SIGNS OF LIFE
    a. The Signs of Life are evidence of the intelligence of life.

19. ORGANIZED MATTER
    a. The material of the body of a "living thing" is organic matter.

20. INNATE INTELLIGENCE
    a. A "living thing" has an inborn intelligence within its body, called Innate Intelligence.

21. THE MISSION OF INNATE INTELLIGENCE
    a. The Mission of Innate Intelligence is to maintain the material of the body of a living thing in active organization.

22. THE QUALITY OF INNATE INTELLIGENCE
    a. There is one hundred per cent of Innate Intelligence in every living thing.

23. THE FUNCTION OF INNATE INTELLIGENCE
    a. The Function of Innate Intelligence is to create adaptive forces to be used in and for the body.
        i. *"Innate Intelligence is the intelligence within the organism, which systematizes the forces already there; it is, scientifically speaking, the principle of organization. Its creations are forces systematized adaptively, and materials built into intelligently planned forms."*[92]

24. THE LIMITS OF ADAPTATION
    a. Innate Intelligence adapts forces and matter for the body as long as it can do so without breaking a universal law.

25. THE CHARACTER OF INNATE FORCES
    a. The forces of Innate never injure or destroy the tissues in which they work.

---

[92] Stephenson, *Chiropractic Textbook*, 262.

i. *"Man cannot build even one tissue cell or repair the same if it is damaged. He may be able to keep a tissue cell alive for a time in artificial surroundings, but the tissue cell merely exists; does not function or do the thing for which it was created, any more than a bear in hibernation shows activity. No, this life shows that it is an adaptable law, able to make instantaneous changes according to environmental conditions of a tissue cell. None but the Creator can change a law, make laws, or circumvent physical laws, so the life current must be a force directly from Law itself."*[93]

26. COMPARISON OF UNIVERSAL AND INNATE FORCES

a. In order to carry on the universal cycle of life, Universal Forces are destructive, and Innate Forces are constructive, as regards structural matter.

27. THE NORMALITY OF INNATE INTELLIGENCE[94]

a. Innate Intelligence is always normal and its function is always normal.

i. *"Intelligence is always perfect—always one hundred per cent. The forces which it assembles are always correct. They are not correct when they reach Tissue Cell if there is interference with transmission, but that is not because of imperfection of Innate's work, but because of the limitations of matter (Prin. 24)."*[95]

ii. *"The imperfection, of course, is in structure. The molecules of a wrecked locomotive are just as good as those in a locomotive in running order, but the*

---

93 Stephenson, *Chiropractic Textbook*, 264.
94 Stephenson, *Chiropractic Textbook*, 269.
95 Stephenson, *Chiropractic Textbook*, 269.

wrecked locomotive is imperfect in structure and therefore is not a good organ to express man's wishes."[96]

28. **THE CONDUCTOR OF MENTAL FORCE**

   a. **The forces of Innate Intelligence operate through or over the nervous system.**

      i. *"Since the nerves are in a cyclic arrangement, this also is not a haphazard arrangement, and they were intended to carry something. Though invisible, that 'something' is more vital than blood.*"[97]

      ii. *"The Spinal Cord is a long cylinder of nerve fibers, surrounding a core of column of gray matter. It is from one-fourth to one-half inch in diameter; about one and one-half ounces in weight, and about eighteen inches in length. It extends from the foramen magnum to the second lumbar vertebra.*"[98]

      iii. *"Transmission is the conduction or conveyance of mental force through or over nerve axons. A properly prepared (created) mental impulse, assembled from the universal supply, is conducted normally by nerve cells. If the mental impulse is one hundred per cent (normal) it does not do the nerve any harm at any time. (Prin. 25.)*"[99]

      iv. *". . . The mental impulse arrives in exactly the same proportions that Innate started it.*"[100]

29. **INTERFERENCE WITH THE TRANSMISSION OF INNATE FORCES**

---

[96] Stephenson, *Chiropractic Textbook*, 269.
[97] Stephenson, *Chiropractic Textbook*, 273.
[98] Stephenson, *Chiropractic Textbook*, 280.
[99] Stephenson, *Chiropractic Textbook*, 290.
[100] Stephenson, *Chiropractic Textbook*, 290.

a. There can be Interference with the Transmission of Innate Forces.

    i. *"The most delicate tissue in the body, nerve tissue, is so sensitive to injury or annoyance that it cannot 'put up' with any rough treatment. It cannot stand pinching or crowding or rough 'shouldering.' Impingement annoys it very much, so that its molecular or its protoplasmic activity is not correct in that case and it does not pass the mental impulse along the length of its axon smoothly—does not let it 'slide through' without loss. No, along its angry or unsound length the mental impulse loses percentage."*[101]

    ii. *"If a nerve is made abnormal in any part (as by impingement) there cannot be normal function of that nerve cell, which is a living organism. The mental impulse is robbed of some of its values and henceforth is (partially or wholly) not a perfectly assembled unit of energies as Innate sent it, but a somewhat dis-sembled unit . . . it is not the perfectly assembled unit that Innate started out on the journey to the cell."*[102]

    iii. *"If the conductor of the current which is conveying the message goes wrong, the message becomes garbled, so that Tissue Cell does not understand it fully."*[103]

30. THE CAUSES OF DIS-EASE

a. Interference with the transmission of Innate forces causes incoordination or dis-ease.

---

[101] Stephenson, *Chiropractic Textbook*, 295.
[102] Stephenson, *Chiropractic Textbook*, 295–296.
[103] Stephenson, *Chiropractic Textbook*, 299.

i. *"Interference with transmission prevents Innate from adapting things universal for use in the body and from coordinating the actions of the tissue cells for the mutual benefit of all cells. Accordingly, the universal forces wear or injure the tissue cells. . . . When a cell is injured, worn down, or 'out of condition,' it is not 'at ease.' Mental force must reach organized matter to make it vibrate properly, that is, live. . . . Mental forces kept from matter cause it to revert to its elemental state."*[104]

ii. *"There is something in a living man that a moment after death is not in the* dead. *The absence of mental force in the body is called* death."[105]

iii. *"Disease is a term used by physicians for sickness. . . . Dis-ease is a Chiropractic term meaning not having ease; or lack of ease."*

iv. *"Trauma is injury to tissues, which impairs or destroys tissue cells but the tissue cells are not sick. In Trauma, tissues are not degenerated or depleted. They are just injured; and this is proven by the fact that a wound will heal readily and healthily, if the region of injury or the body is not dis-eased."*[106]

v. *"FORAMEN. 'A small opening, perforation, or orifice.'"*

vi. *"The spinal nerve does not completely fill the foramen, which also contains blood vessels, fat and areolar tissue."*

104 Stephenson, *Chiropractic Textbook*, 301.
105 Stephenson, *Chiropractic Textbook*, 301–302.
106 Stephenson, *Chiropractic Textbook*, 302.

vii. *"Owing to the movability of the vertebrae and the possibility of the vertebrae becoming subluxated, an abnormal change in the size or shape of the foramen will cause the nerve to be impinged, if not actually pressed or pinched."*[107]

viii. *"IMPINGEMENT: 'To encroach or infringe (on or upon)."*[108]

ix. *"When the body walls of the foramen are out of their normal positions, they crowd upon the contents of the foramen, which in turn crowd upon one or more axons in the spinal nerve. Since nerve cells are extremely delicate, very little pressure is necessary to disarrange its working capacity to some extent."*

x. *"Being very delicate, constant pressure, hourly or daily encroachments, even if not constant, will annoy this very sensitive tissue cell."*

xi. *"An annoyed or sick nerve cannot conduct properly."*[109]

31. <u>SUBLUXATIONS, THE PHYSICAL REPRESENTATIVE OF THE CAUSE OF DIS-EASE</u>

a. Interference with transmission, in the body, is always directly or indirectly due to subluxations in the spinal column.

i. *"A Vertebra is in its normal position when it is in proper juxtaposition with the vertebra above and the one below, when all its articulations are in proper apposition; and so that it does not*

---

107 Stephenson, *Chiropractic Textbook*, 303.
108 Stephenson, *Chiropractic Textbook*, 303.
109 Stephenson, *Chiropractic Textbook*, 304.

impinge nerves and interfere with the transmission of mental impulses."[110]

    ii.   "*A Subluxation is the result of unbalanced resistive forces in response to an invading penetrative force.*"[111]

    iii.   "*External Forces are environmental or universal or physical forces; forces not assembled by Innate Intelligence.*"[112]

    iv.   "*Penetrative Forces are invasive forces; forces external which force their way into the body, and their effects upon tissue, in spite of Innate's resistance. Or, they are forces in the body which Innate does not desire, and which she tries to expel; or to prevent their action. They are in numerous forms; as physical, chemical, and mechanical.*"[113]

    v.   "*INTERNAL FORCES. Forces made my Innate. They are for use in and for the body. They are universal forces assembled or adapted for use in the body. They are for adaptation to other universal forces.*"[114]

32. <u>COORDINATION</u>[115]

    a.   Coordination is the principle of harmonious action of all the parts of an organism, in fulfilling their offices or purposes.

33. <u>THE LAW OF DEMAND AND SUPPLY</u>[116]

---

[110] Stephenson, *Chiropractic Textbook*, 312.
[111] Stephenson, *Chiropractic Textbook*, 322.
[112] Stephenson, *Chiropractic Textbook*, 325.
[113] Stephenson, *Chiropractic Textbook*, 326.
[114] Stephenson, *Chiropractic Textbook*, 327.
[115] Stephenson, *Chiropractic Textbook*, 331.
[116] Stephenson, *Chiropractic Textbook*, 333.

a. The Law of Demand and Supply is existent in the body in its ideal state; wherein the "clearing house" is the brain, Innate the virtuous "banker," brain cells "clerks," and nerve cells "messengers."

About the Author

Dr. Steve Judson is a chiropractic educator and trainer and one of the top speakers at chiropractic seminars and health events around the world. Dr. Judson's passion is to help humans heal from within, unleash their innate healing power, and reach their fullest potential through chiropractic.

Since 2002, Dr. Judson has practiced chiropractic in Newington, Connecticut, where he is the owner and operator of one of the largest chiropractic facilities in the United States. As an upper cervical specialist and a trainer of chiropractors, Dr. Judson preaches and practices a hardcore, pull-no-punches approach to human health focused around a single, burning question: "How's Your Atlas?" He travels the world educating doctors and patients about the human body's innate wisdom to heal itself via the central nervous system, and the supreme importance of the atlas bone (the first cervical vertebra). His movement, "Wake Up, Humans," is devoted to helping men, women, and children discover their destinies and unlock the incredible healing power inherent within every human body.

Dr. Judson's mission has taken him around the world—to Russia, Central America, Tobago, and the Dominican Republic. His books, *Wake Up, Humans!* and *Atlas Adjusted* are tools designed to spread the message of the chiropractic principle and its ability to manifest ultimate human abundance. His greatest source of pride is his incredible family: his wife Tammy and their five beautiful children, Kylie, Sierra, Brooke, Kane and Jaimee.

Made in the USA
Middletown, DE
24 December 2019